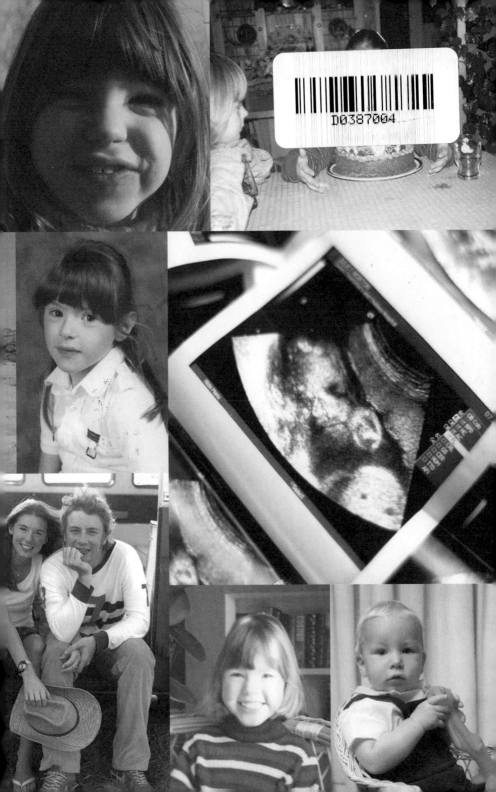

Jools Oliver

THE DIARY OF AN HONEST MUM

Jools Oliver

THE DIARY OF AN HONEST MUM

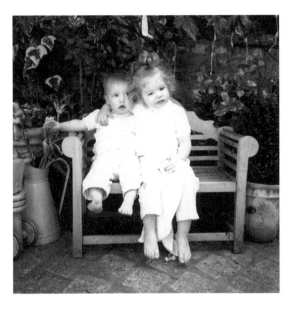

HYPERION

NEW YORK

Note to Reader: Please note this book contains a personal account of pregnancy and is not intended to replace professional medical advice. All matters regarding your health and pregnancy require medical supervision. Consult your physician before adopting the suggestions in this book. Neither this nor any other related book mentioned should be used as a substitute for qualified medical care and treatment. The author and publisher disclaim any liability directly or indirectly from the use of the material in this book.

Photographs by Jamie Oliver MBE (well, it's got to be used sometimes!) and Chris Terry. Additional photos by Dave Bennett / Getty Images (page 57), John Carey (pages 84-85), Harry Borden (pages 171 and 178), and David Loftus (page 211).

ISBN: 1-4013-0270-X

Hyperion books are available for special promotions and premiums. For details contact Michael Rentas, Assistant Director, Inventory Operations, Hyperion, 77 West 66th Street, 12th floor, New York, New York 10023, or call 212-456-0133.

First U.S. Edition

10 9 8 7 6 5 4 3 2 1

CONTENTS

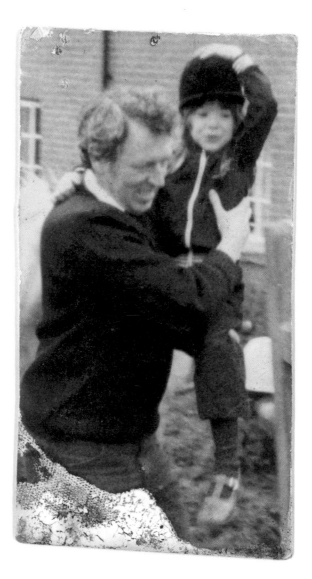

To my wonderful dad, who I know has been with
me all the way. Without him watching over me I would
never have achieved my goal of writing this book.

To my gorgeous, patient, supportive, fantastic husband, Jamie.

To my two precious and adorable girls, Poppy and Daisy—
the reason I was able to write this book in the first place.

To my amazing mum, for always being there for me and
my girls, and for listening patiently when I was writing.

To my two fab sisters, Nathalie and Lisa, who deserve the best.

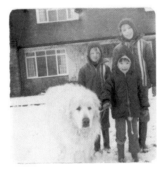

Jools Oliver lives with her husband and two little girls
in London and Essex. This is her first book.

INTRODUCTION

The Diary of an Honest Mum is about a life-changing experience, and one that all women who are pregnant for the first time will go through. Not everyone's experience is the same and this book is my own take on things, but I hope that I might be of some help to you when you're going through the same worries that I had as a new mum. And even if you're not pregnant at the moment, I hope you might just enjoy reading it anyway.

I have to admit that it has always been a secret passion of mine to write a book. When I became pregnant for the first time and started out on the incredible journey to becoming a mum, the experiences that I was going through – the worries, the never-ending excitement, the miracles, the laughter and the mind-blowing hard work – really stretched and challenged me in ways that I never expected. And we've only been parents for three years! So I thought that it would be fun to write about the journey I found myself on.

This certainly hasn't been written as a guidebook for pregnant women, or as a medical reference book for that matter, although I have included a glossary of medical terms at the back of the book. When I first discovered I was pregnant, I found it very hard to find one book that encompassed everything that I was interested in knowing about. I wanted to have a bit of medical stuff, set out simply with all the obvious questions and answers, and I also wanted a bit about the aftercare of your newborn (although I found it hard to even think past the labor!). And I wanted all this to be bound up with a lot of humor, because with everything being thrown at you, you will definitely need a laugh! So this book is my honest look at what happened to me and all the experiences I went through, from trying to get pregnant to having my second daughter a year after my first. Whether you're trying for a baby, pregnant for the first time or bringing up two children under two (like I was last year) then I hope this book might help to show you how I coped in those circumstances.

The way I have set out the book will show you everything that happened to me from "minus nine" (when I became pregnant) to "one" (when Poppy had her first birthday) and is really my personal journal. Towards the end of the book there is a section called "The Food Bit" which, being married to Jamie, I couldn't really leave out, as food is such an important issue in our family! It's a handful of recipes that I make to feed the girls now they are both on solids and hopefully it will help to give you some ideas in the kitchen if you are stuck.

This is simply my story. I hope that you can relate to it in some way, that you enjoy it and maybe, if you have time, even relax with it in the bath!

PROLOGUE

So here I am on my knees surrounded by antibacterial wipes, disinfectant spray and POO! A very familiar scene to mums of young children all over the world, I'm sure. When I first became pregnant I would daydream about how wonderful it would be to be a mum – I wasn't really thinking of how baby wipes would become my best friend in moments like this. . . .

Once again my youngest daughter, Daisy (who will no doubt kill me for telling you this story in 10 years' time!), has decided to cover herself in her poo. This has been happening on a regular basis for the last few weeks. She decides to wait until she is inside her freshly laundered Grobag, in her pristine white cot, surrounded with toys and books, during her lunchtime nap. And then she poos. And then she gets it EVERYWHERE, usually decorating her cot with it. I generally never make it in time to catch her. I walk into her room and see her cheeky smile as she shows off her artistic abilities and invites me to join in!

Today it doesn't seem at all funny though. I am a bit ticked off as I see that she has done it yet again. I'm tired. We've just moved to a new house and the place is full of builders, plumbers and engineers. All I can hear are drills and the pounding of the radio, and I've got a headache. We're now going to be very late for Poppy's ballet class and on top of all this the plumbers have turned off the water and electricity . . . arghhhhhhh!

So as I said, I am now on my knees wondering what or who to scrub first. I've got Daisy running naked around the bathroom, still covered in poo, and Poppy now awake and dragging her dolls, books and blankets into the bath. I decide to tackle the one object which is stationary, and also the worst affected . . . in this case it happens to be Buzz Lightyear! How on earth Daisy managed to get poo stuck between his head and his helmet I will never know. Putting on a pair of surgical gloves, I attempt to give Buzz back some of his dignity, but at the crucial moment (I accidentally pressed a button) he announced, "THIS IS AN INTERGALACTIC EMERGENCY!" You said it, Buzz. I didn't know whether to laugh or cry. . . . Welcome to motherhood!

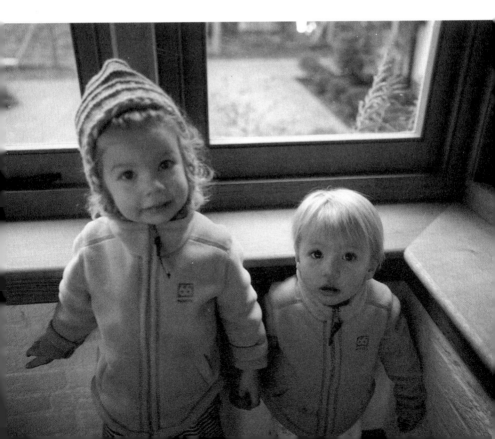

CHAPTER ONE

Getting to Minus Nine ...

I have always wanted children since before I can remember.
Like most little girls, I knew all the names of my children
and of course their sexes! Ironically, I really wanted to have
four boys . . . I am not sure why. Perhaps it was because I was
a complete tomboy up until the age of 15, most of my friends
were boys, I supported Arsenal football team (because my
dad did and I was a daddy's girl!) and wore Doc Martens
boots with everything. I knew that family was also very
important to Jamie, and we started talking about children
very early on in our relationship. Once we were married we
would start trying for children straightaway.

So with this in mind, we decided to get married when
we did (I was 26 and Jamie was 25). I started to take folic acid
to prepare my body and read up about pregnancy. I couldn't
wait . . . Trying for a baby is brilliant fun, of course, until you
realize that maybe it's taking slightly longer to get pregnant
than you first imagined. I naively thought that I would
definitely have a honeymoon baby and it would all be very
simple and romantic. How wrong was I?

I had always known about my possible problems with
fertility because I'd had irregular periods from about the age
of 16, and had been to see the doctor. He had confirmed that
I had polycystic ovaries and that there was a chance they
may cause me problems later in life. But we had purposely

pushed it out of our minds, hoping that doing all the textbook things would be enough to conceive. I even bought a batch of pregnancy test kits when I returned home from our honeymoon (thinking that we had definitely made a baby). If you have ever found yourself in this position you'll understand when I say that trying just one test is never enough. They all tested negative.

The weeks went by and there was no sign of my period (although this was not unusual for me) so I took this to mean that I WAS pregnant and the negative testing was wrong. I then decided to try out different brands of pregnancy tests, as I was convinced that just being 99% accurate was not enough. Of course I hid them all from Jamie and took them secretly, fantasizing that I would emerge from the bathroom and come downstairs to him with those two wonderful words, "I'm pregnant!"

One night I remember really craving strawberry cheesecake. I just had to have some and, as I didn't have any at home, it became an obsession. Jamie was at work, it was 8:30 pm and I couldn't think of anything else, so I hopped into the car and drove to our local Sainsbury's for an individual cheesecake. Naturally I took this to be the start of my pregnancy cravings! However, I wasn't pregnant. This process went on for a number of months, and in between the trying to conceive and the tests it seemed to consume my life.

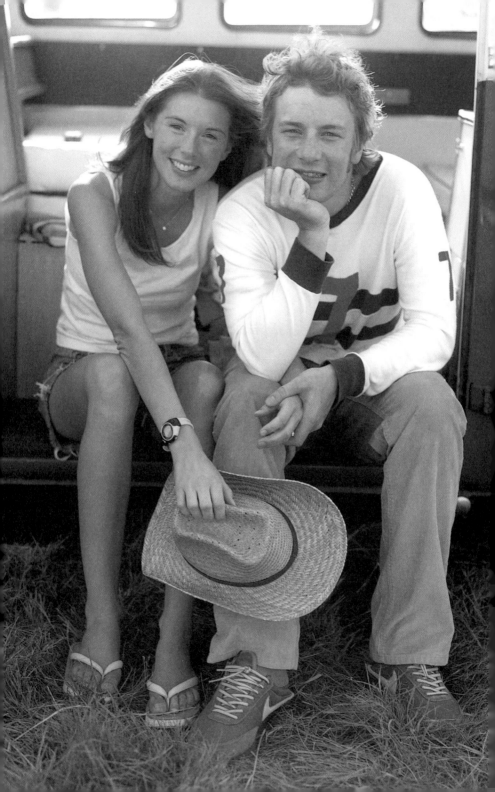

HOW TO CONCEIVE THE OLIVER WAY!

It was with a heavy heart that each month went by. Despite all my hopes that I was pregnant, I would feel the familiar "drag" of an oncoming period. It's very hard to explain this part of our story as it is so personal, but quite frankly (without going into *too* much detail) it's a part which is worth telling just for the laughs!

Let me start by going back in time a bit. A few months before our wedding, I was out of work. I had been working as a television researcher at the BBC and my contract had finished. Not being sure if I wanted to pursue this career path any further, I decided to wait a while until I had sorted myself out. It was then that Jamie asked if I wanted to become his PA (I just find this whole notion hilarious now that I think back to it!). I agreed, as it meant that I would get to see him every day and I thought it would be fun, plus I was never really a career girl anyway – who was I kidding? – I wanted the babies, the baking and the roses around the door!

So, I set about learning to become Jamie's ever-so-efficient PA. At the time, his first series of *The Naked Chef* had just been televised and he was slowly gaining notoriety. He had been organizing his entire diary in a little battered notepad with various scribbles about meetings and appointments, so I decided the first thing to do was to organize everything. Now, for me that meant spending a hell of a lot of money in Rymans stationers on brightly colored stickers and charts, exotic-looking pens and multi-colored drawing pins! I organized a small office space in the hallway of our one-

bedroom flat in West Hampstead and set out a wall chart
of his day-to-day meetings. It looked fab and took all of,
hmmm, one day. . . . What was I to do now? I didn't have a clue
about being a PA. It seemed to me that all it involved was
tidying the office-cum-hallway, doing food shopping and then
using the phone to, well, chat to my friends. It was obvious
that I was not cut out for this business. Plus, I never saw
Jamie – as promised and outlined by him in the job spec(!). I
was also getting fed up with constantly fielding calls from a
persistent journalist who wanted Jamie to pose naked, but for
a few strategically placed grapes, for the centerfold of a girls'
mag. Well, I can tell you now, NO WAY! So I was fired. My
office chair was pulled abruptly from underneath my bum
and I was quickly replaced by my best friend, Nicola, who had
a lot of professional PA skills behind her. This was actually
even better for me now because when Nix called to speak to
Jamie on a professional level, I was there to field the calls and
talk girls' gossip first, so everyone was happy.

You're probably wondering why I'm even telling you this
story, so let me get on with it. Way back then, before I
realized there was a possibility of fertility problems, I used to
label my fertile days on the giant, newly erected wall chart in
my office. The good days for a bit of lovin' were labeled in red
ink just above whichever meeting with the BBC or
appointment with the accountant Jamie had on that day.
There it was in red and white, much to Jamie's annoyance,
for all to see! Of course, when I was made redundant (I
prefer to say that actually, as "fired" sounds so harsh), my
wall chart became obsolete, so it was left to me and Nix to

organize my fertile days to correspond with Jamie's book meetings or filming days. Thank God she was my best friend, as I couldn't have revealed these sorts of details to just anyone at the time!

As time went on it became obvious that these little private "fertility" meetings that Jamie and I were having during the day were not amounting to anything, if you know what I mean. So it was at that point that we had to admit temporary defeat and seek professional help and possible medical intervention. This was the situation I had been dreading.

Throughout this time my mum had been my constant support. We're really close to each other, and it's not unusual for me to call her at least five or six times a day. Jamie finds this unbelievable – he can't work out what I have left to say to Mum after the fifth time we have spoken. This is true of both my sisters, Lisa and Nathalie, as well. It is a wonder Mum has time to function during a normal day without her phone attached to her ear like a telephone assistance operator!

I HATE hospitals and even doctors' offices for that matter, because I don't like to admit that I might be ill or need help. I like everything around me to be sunny and bright and I hate confrontation or drastic changes (ironic really when I am the world's worst hypochondriac). The only people I could open up to about such private things are Jamie and my mum and sisters, so taking the first step in going to see a doctor was confirmation that all was not right with Juliette Oliver.

As it goes, a simple visit to my GP was all that was required at first. I explained to him the problems we seemed to be having in conceiving and about my polycystic ovaries.

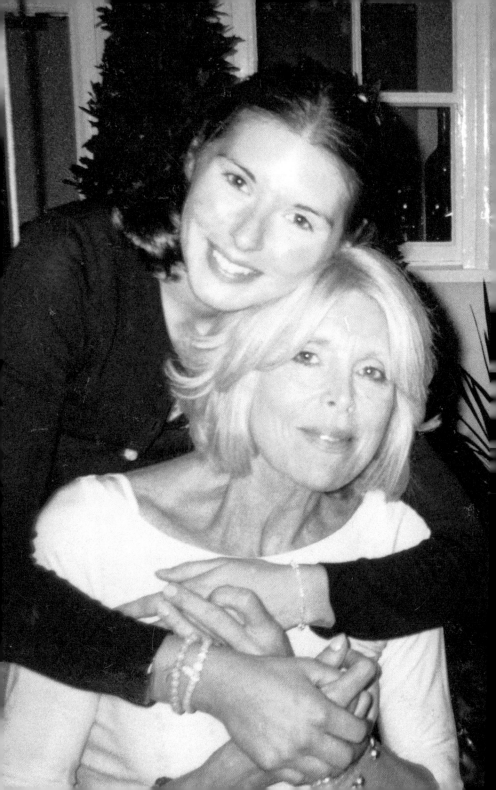

He immediately gave me a referral letter to see Mr. Geoffrey Trew, whom he considered to be the best fertility doctor in Britain. He worked as part of the team at the Queen Charlotte and Chelsea Hospital in Hammersmith, under the guidance of Sir Robert Winston.

The first stage was over and I felt relieved, but of course this was only the beginning. . . .

We booked our first appointment with Mr. Trew, but as he had such a great reputation, he was booked so far in advance that we had to wait two months before we could see him. I was counting the days until the visit to the hospital with anticipation, nerves and total excitement.

It turned into one of the most stressful journeys of my life – not only had I gone to the wrong hospital, but Jamie was running late after having gotten stuck at work and he was negotiating the traffic on his moped only to find that he, too, was in the wrong part of town. I drove towards the right hospital, through the rush-hour traffic, tears streaming down my face, completely convinced that we had missed our slot. Then I saw Jamie on his moped, wearing his egg-shaped helmet, weaving in and out of the smoky traffic jam. He managed to arrive way before me and was not the least bit stressed (that's the big difference between the two of us!). We had made it, but were an hour late and I was a weeping mess. As soon as we entered Mr. Trew's office, a feeling of complete calm and positivity washed over me. I knew that this man was going to help us achieve our dream.

Having ascertained that we were both perfectly healthy, he thought that perhaps one of us had a medical hiccup that was hindering our efforts to conceive. I knew that it was probably me, due to my past medical history and polycystic ovaries, but Mr. Trew insisted that Jamie have the rudimentary checks and investigations – just in case (much to Jamie's dismay . . . what is it about men and their sperm?).

I was given three basic checks:

* A simple blood test to assess my hormone levels.
* Something called a trans-vaginal ultrasound to look at my ovaries and womb.
* An X-ray, called a hysterosalpingogram (or HSG), to check that everything in the womb was all working correctly and that my "tubes" were healthy.

And all Jamie had to do was have a sample of his sperm analyzed – hmmm, easier said than done!

At home that night I began to worry. I just couldn't stop thinking about what it all meant. I had no idea that there could possibly be so many reasons as to why we were not conceiving. Even more scary was the thought that all the results could show that everything was fine. What happened then? Would we be considered lost causes? It had all become a bit too daunting.

For Jamie, the only thing to do was to be positive. He was convinced that everything would be fine, and so set about arranging his little "test." Now, Jamie being Jamie, he insisted on completing his task in the comfort and safety of our own home, rather than in the clinical surroundings of the hospital, but this posed a few problems. The main one being that (and now I'm getting clinical!) a man's semen sample has to be as fresh as possible in order to get an accurate result. So, after a few phone calls to the medical team, we worked out that if he made his sample at home he would need a courier to be waiting outside to take it from Hampstead to Hammersmith in under 15 minutes – as if this baby-making process wasn't stressful enough!

Deciding against a courier (the London courier system didn't fill me with the utmost confidence), Jamie decided he would take it there himself on his moped.

With the deed done, he hopped on his bike and rode off into the distance in a scene reminiscent of *The Dukes of Hazzard*. If only people had known what he had tucked under his waterproof jacket!

On arrival at the hospital, with minutes to spare, he raced to the samples department, remembering to keep his helmet on in case (God forbid) anyone should recognize him. When he reached the counter, he handed his sample to a very friendly woman. She held the little see-through bottle in her hand and, as Jamie skulked away, she called him back by shouting at him down the hallway. Reluctantly and subserviently Jamie went back over to her. She peered over her glasses and promptly asked him to remove his helmet. "Excuse me, are you who I think you are? Are you THE Jamie Oliver, as in Jamie Oliver the Naked Chef?" Well, you can imagine how absolutely embarrassed he was. But it didn't stop there. As she called a few of her staff members to come and gawk at The Naked Chef HIMSELF she proceeded to toss – yes, toss Jamie's sperm from one hand to the other, excitedly expressing her passion for his food and his program, which happened to have aired the night before . . . bloody classic! It was probably the only time Jamie has ever turned totally red and wanted the ground to swallow him up. He told me later that he truly had never been so embarrassed in all his life. I, on the other hand, almost wet myself laughing when I heard the story. A little bit of light relief (if you know what I mean!) was just what the doctor had ordered.

Compared to Jamie's experience, my tests went along very smoothly. On our second visit to see Mr. Trew, we went through the results. I was very nervous because whatever he said would decide our fate. First, it showed that my hormone level was normal . . . check. And my trans-vaginal showed that my polycystic ovaries were still there, as we suspected, but showed no abnormality so, okay . . . half a check. My hysterosalpingogram showed a normal uterine cavity (whatever that is) but there was a problem at the end of both my fallopian tubes. A dye had been inserted into my womb during the test and it had filled the whole length of the tubes, but not managed to come out the other end. So there was some sort of obstruction. The next step was to further investigate the problem by having what is called a laparoscopy – a simple operation to see inside the abdomen (by passing a camera through a small cut in the abdominal wall).

I was now beside myself with worry. Not only did I have a phobia about operations and being under anaesthesia, but it was beginning to get serious, and for me there was no going back.

However, there was no need to worry. The procedure was painless and the results were surprisingly encouraging. My fallopian tubes were just stuck underneath my ovaries –

it was simply a process of freeing them up and finding that they were still perfectly healthy . . . excellent, fantastic, brilliant news! We were relieved beyond belief, and I finally allowed myself a little bit of hope.

With all the investigations complete, we were ready to move forward. The first thing was to get my periods on track and on a regular cycle – something I've actually never had. This was achieved by taking some tablets called Provera. They immediately allowed me to have a regular, normal period – it was amazing. After all these years I was starting to feel like a real woman. Once that was established, it was on to a drug called Clomid that is used to treat infertility when women have problems ovulating. Mr. Trew gave me a three-month supply and I started on a low dose. During this time I was constantly monitored.

I had to make continuous trips to the hospital for various tests because when you start taking Clomid you have to be prepared to go through a hell of a lot of monitoring. I felt that if it meant I'd be one step closer to conceiving a baby, then it was just fine. The tests were there to make sure that I was getting the desired effect from the Clomid – that I was producing either one or two eggs, as opposed to none at all or too many (ironically!). The way they checked this was through a process called follicle tracking, and it involved several blood tests and scans focused on the development of my eggs and ovaries. I had become a human pincushion overnight. Even Jamie stopped accompanying me on these visits, as there was only so much he could take of the "needle in the arm trick." I was starting to get fed up seeing his feet tucked behind the hospital curtains as he hid behind the screens. Giving me reassurance from across the room wasn't quite the same as holding my hand – I became so used to it that the nurses and I would have a laugh at my husband's expense! These follicle-tracking checks lasted for a couple of months – when they start to show good ovulation the tracking is ceased for months.

Unfortunately for me, Clomid wasn't the most enjoyable drug to be on and I suffered from side effects, such as dizziness, hot sweats and nausea. For the first couple of weeks I felt fine but as time went on, and the pressures at home increased, it all took its toll.

We had just managed to buy a maisonette in Hampstead. It was our dream one-bedroom house with our own front door – something which we had never had before. I was so excited – this was a brand-new setting for our married life and, hopefully, a family. But the renovations were not finished on time (how shocking!) and so it meant we had to move into temporary accommodations. We were very lucky as, at the time, Jamie was working at Monte's Restaurant, which had living quarters attached, so we stayed there. Jamie worked in the evenings downstairs in the restaurant – it wasn't ideal as it was a bit of an upheaval but it was incredibly convenient.

I had started to get little dizzy spells that weren't a problem at first, but as they increased it got a bit scary. These spells came only at certain times – notably when I was in public or put into a situation where I felt slightly uncomfortable. As time moved on, the dizzy spells were coupled with hot sweats, nausea and feelings that I was going to faint. I hated these sensations. They were so consuming and left me exhausted and upset. It wasn't long before I realized that these episodes were actually panic attacks brought on, possibly, by the Clomid, coupled with the stress that I'd been under for the last couple of months. It built up so badly that even a simple trip to a department store was hell.

One day Jamie and I went along to have a look around Harrods, as it was fairly close to where we were staying. It should have been fun but I only managed to get to the first floor before rushing out in a flood of tears, alarmed that I was enclosed in an environment with hundreds of people and no obvious exit. What was wrong with me? I had never had this problem before. I had always been shy, but I loved going out and having fun, and a shopping trip like that would normally have filled me with pure joy, not terror!

Okay, I thought, it was time for me to take stock and, just at the right time, Jamie announced that he was going on a three-week tour to Australia and suggested that, for once, I stop worrying about flying and go with him. It was just what I needed – time away with Jamie and something exciting to look forward to. As much as I HATED flying, I certainly wasn't prepared to waste another month on Clomid without Jamie around. After all, I didn't think conceiving a child with my husband on the opposite side of the world would be all that easy!

With something else to think about, all the anxiety about trying to have a baby was pushed to the back of my mind – although I had decided to pack those little fertility sticks (you pee on them and they tell you when it's your best time to have sex). I had used these before in the past, but as my periods had never been regular, they were almost pointless. Now on the Clomid at least I knew when I was going to have one and, in turn, could just about predict when I was going to be most fertile.

The trip was fantastic, especially as Nicola, Jamie's PA, was along for the trip, as well as another lovely friend of mine, Pia. We stayed in Melbourne and had the time of our lives. It was certainly one trip that I'll never forget (as I was later to discover in more ways than one!).

On the last leg of the tour, we were to fly out to New Zealand – for this part of the trip it was just me, Jamie and his agent. I saw this as our chance to spend some quality time together (or so I thought). However, for those last four days Jamie was as hectic as ever, but I didn't care because we were staying in a beautiful hotel looking out over the water and the weather was fantastic. I spent most of the time splayed out on the balcony ordering room service and reading mags!

Of course, during this time Jamie and I were trying for the baby. As you can imagine, and most probably know if you've been in a similar situation, some of the magic captured during making love can be lost when you are checking flow charts and peeing on pink sticks before each session. (You must excuse me for the next few paragraphs. I may revert to a slightly corny mode of writing as my mum and mum-in-law will no doubt read this and, frankly, using the words "shag" and "sex" might upset them, so there will be the odd "making love" or "bonk" in here. Jamie, turn away now!)

I was your typical dominant, hyper, over-organized mother-in-the-making! I am not quite sure how Jamie put up with my behavior. I was demanding you-know-what at the oddest times

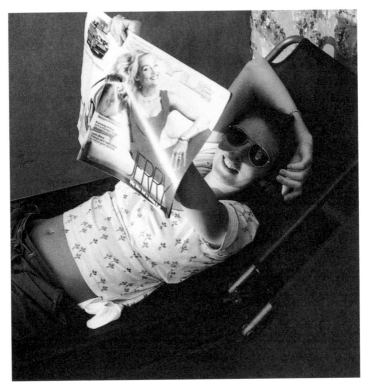

of the day, due to what my fertility sticks said, and in the most inconvenient places. Poor boy – he must have been exhausted. On one such occasion he had to film a commercial out in the New Zealand countryside, which meant he had to be up at 4:00 am to leave with the rest of the crew. ... Believe me, sex was the last thing on my mind, too, but I pinned Jamie down and before he knew it (it didn't take long!) he was sharing an elevator down to the car with his agent looking, ahem, how can I put it ... disheveled and exhausted!

I didn't look too much better myself. I decided that it was in my best interests to maneuver myself into my usual postcoital position of legs in the air, resting against the wall and lying on the bed. Thank God for on-demand movies in hotel rooms. I watched *Coyote Ugly* in this position a couple of times until the sun came up about three hours later!

So there I was hoping secretly that my acrobatics had reserved me a place in the line of mothers-to-be. We were flying home that afternoon. I was so excited, as we were going to be moving into our new little house as soon as we got back, hopefully putting the last couple of months behind us. Before we left for our late-afternoon flight, I did a quick impromptu wee stick check – oh my God, it was hot pink and I was still fertile. In fact, even more so than I had been last night. We had no time to lose . . . here we go again. But it was too late and we would have missed our flight if we had had that little extra, so there was nothing but to go to the airport. I was frantically trying to work out my fertile dates with changing time zones – the only thing left to do was join the Mile High Club! But with Jamie's agent in tow, that wasn't going to be an option. Plus, have you seen the size of airplane bathrooms?! Fretting for seven hours, we reached our stopover in LA. While most passengers relaxed in the lounge having a drink, we wandered around aimlessly to see if we could find a little cubicle with a bed that we could use. I was sure they had them there – this was LA for God's sake. Didn't businessmen need to catch a few winks and a shower before they embarked on the next leg of their journey, and didn't panicking fertile women need a bed so they could contribute to the world with a little light breeding? I mean, this is the 21st century!

By now I had almost given up, convinced we had missed our

window of opportunity. Even Jamie's agent was joining the search party – how embarrassing for an agent, trying to find a bed in an airport so a client and his wife could have a bonk! Well, unfortunately, we didn't manage to find one anywhere, so it was homeward bound on the next leg of the flight.

As I sat there on the flight to London, I was convinced that I had missed my window of baby opportunity. My disappointment couldn't be hidden. Just before the seat belt sign was lit for landing, I gave myself just one last chance on the fertility stick . . . and, by goodness, I was still in the running. The look on Jamie's face when I came beaming out of the airplane bathroom was quite a picture – I'm sure he was thinking the samething as me but with a hell of a lot less enthusiasm!

There is just one last part of this Benny Hill charade left to tell. We only had a few fertile hours to go before this second opportunity passed us by again, so we asked our taxi driver to speed like lightning to get us home from Heathrow in time for another quick go.

We were supposed to move into our new house that day (well, actually, it was a flat with stairs, but it felt so grown up!), and during a quick call to my sister Lisa, who was managing the project and the contractors, she told us that (as we suspected) the house was totally unfinished and full of strapping tabloid-reading, pork-pie-eating, tea-with-10-sugars-drinking BUILDERS. This was certainly not the ideal situation to conceive a child in! But, as my mum would say, the Norton sisters get the job done and so, with a little forceful instruction and a touch of bossiness, Lisa had the contractors putting together our flat-packed iron bed while she got out some fresh sheets and prepared the room for us.

Like a scene from *Trading Spaces*, Lisa had the bedroom completely sorted and the workers banished to the pub up the road (confused but NOT complaining!) by the time we got there. Arriving at the house, Jamie gallantly carried me over the threshold – maybe this was going to be romantic after all! Perhaps the least romantic thing about this whole farcical scene was when Jamie and I emerged victorious (as you do) from the house and walked into Hampstead. We passed the pub where the workers and my sister were ensconced over their pints. They looked up sheepishly as we arrived (well, about as sheepishly as they could) and it was VERY obvious that the cat was out of the bag as they offered us a drink. Judging by their faces and sniggers, I expected them to burst into applause like in a movie, with the whole pub joining in as well. Thank God we were spared that little embarrassment; nonetheless I left the pub a slightly darker shade of maroon and so did Jamie!

So, with all of these different episodes, it's hard to think which was the "magic" one that sent us our baby. Personally, I like to think that Poppy was conceived on our vacation in Italy, which we took the day after we came home from Australia. We stayed at the same hotel in which we had spent our honeymoon the year before; on this occasion I slipped in a quick visit to a little church perched high in the mountains and said a little prayer. Who knows? But I can tell you that the whole process of conception was one hell of a journey, in more ways than one!

DISCOVERING I WAS PREGNANT WITH POPPY

I am sure everyone remembers vividly where they were when they did that amazing pregnancy test – the one where two blue lines show instead of just the one. It can be such a shock. Especially when you have been used to sitting on the toilet (like me) for the millionth time, your bum numb, willing the second blue line to appear as if by magic!

Well, this is how it happened for me. It was an ordinary day in the Oliver household. Jamie had gone off to film a Sainsbury's ad and I was settling into life in the new house.

After returning from Italy, I had been unpacking and organizing our new home for a week and felt exhausted. I planned to sort out our wardrobe and had set aside the whole day to be surrounded by Jamie's muddy sneakers and my mismatched underwear – no easy task!

It was about the time in the month for my period to start if I had been unsuccessful in conceiving with the prescribed medication. I had been taking the Clomid now for three months and was expecting my period like clockwork. It was July 4 – American Independence Day and the day of Madonna's "Blond Ambition" tour at Wembley. (I know this as I had eagerly awaited tickets!) The three-month cycle of tablets had run their course so I was expecting to re-evaluate the situation with my doctor and perhaps think about moving on to a stronger form of fertility treatment. I was convinced that I should give Clomid one more month and had planned to call the wonderful Mr. Trew that day and ask for some more.

While running my usual morning bath I was rummaging

through the as yet unpacked box labeled "bath stuff" looking for a scrubbing brush when I came across one solitary and very lonely looking pregnancy test . . . I just had to use it up. "I'll buy another batch of 10 when I go shopping next," I thought. Little did I know!

It was done like any other test. I read the instructions (that was certainly more out of habit than necessity), peed on the stick and waited. This time I decided to take the test into the bedroom and ever so casually watch *This Morning*. With one eye on Richard and Judy, I glanced at the test. This time it was different – there before my eyes the test became positive! That magical blue line appeared and I just didn't believe it. I thought that it couldn't be true. I started to shake and I literally felt weak at the knees. I grabbed the phone to call Jamie but his bloody phone was turned off! I had to tell someone, so I called my mum – I screamed into her answering machine, "I'M PREGNANT! I'M PREGNANT! I'M PREGNANT!" That certainly got her out of the bath! Next was to tell Jamie – not so easy as he was in the middle of filming and I had to get through about five people before I actually spoke to him. Even then I was screaming down the phone with excitement – of course he was unable to show a reaction as the room was filled with people, but I could tell by his voice that he was brimming with excitement.

As any woman who finds herself pregnant for the first time will tell you, a positive result will not let you rest. I found myself constantly checking the line just to reassure myself . . . and I did this every hour!

The next thing for me to do was to ring the lovely Mr. Trew and tell him my news. "How fantastic is this?" I thought, as just

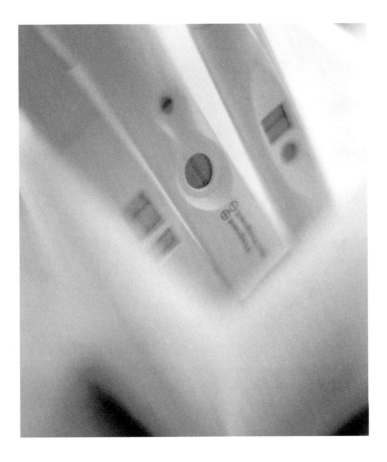

an hour ago I was about to call him for a very different reason!

With my head firmly in the clouds I relayed the whole mini-saga to Mr. Trew (whether he wanted all the details or not!). As with all good doctors, he answered all my questions no matter how crazy they sounded and, believe me, they ranged from the sublime to the absolutely ridiculous! This was to be the first of many telephone calls I made to the poor doctor on a regular basis throughout the nine months and beyond. But each question and comment was taken with real compassion, patience and sensitivity, which makes me think that I am not the only newly pregnant mum to stalk her gynecologist!

With a normal, straightforward pregnancy it is likely that once your GP has confirmed that you are pregnant it is simply a matter of waiting until your three-month check where hopefully all the fun begins and your baby becomes more of a reality. But in my case, and with my fertility problems, it was not as clear-cut as that. As soon as I had made that initial call to Mr. Trew, I had to make my way down to the hospital where I had all my preliminary tests carried out. Not content with just telling Jamie our news on the phone, I couldn't resist popping in to see him on the way to the hospital. I was clutching the pregnancy test in my hand and attempted to discreetly coax Jamie out of his meeting. I'm sure those who were there noticed that something big was up between us.

The rest of the day I was perched on cloud nine. I couldn't wait for Jamie to come home so we could discuss our baby and dream about what it was going to be like to be parents.

It was a really hot day so when I got back from the hospital I got into my holiday shorts (basically, the shorts that should only be saved for the beach as they were too short and too tight!) and a bright pink vest. I felt fantastic, but obviously my hormones had kicked in and my fashion sense had been sent awry! I went to my favorite place in Hampstead – Burgh House – which is a gorgeous National Trust house that serves the best twice-baked potatoes. I wondered if the waiter knew that I was pregnant. I wondered if anyone could tell for that matter. Perhaps my incessant questioning regarding the cheese on my potato being pasteurized or not was enough for the waiter to think that I was either mad or warming a bun in the oven. It tasted like one of the best meals I have ever had. And of course I had taken my pregnancy test with me in my bag and every so often I checked for those two blue lines.

I still have THAT pregnancy test for Poppy along with the three positive tests that I took for my second baby, Daisy, in a special box and, yes, the lines are still there – just like magic!

CHAPTER TWO

The First Trimester

QUESTIONS, QUESTIONS, QUESTIONS

I couldn't get used to being pregnant. The thought that
there was a little human being the size of a rice grain curled
up inside me was unbelievable!

I became obsessed with those charts that you can use to tell
you what stage your pregnancy is at. I loved visualizing what my
baby might look like. Over and over again I would read about the
development of my baby according to how many weeks
pregnant I was. I drove Jamie mad as, on many of his kitchen
work surfaces and, of course, the fridge, I pinned due date charts
(brilliant when you are trying to work out what possible star sign
your baby might be), development charts and ideas for names
(and I was only seven weeks pregnant at this point!).

Naturally, my new obsession did not stop there. Gone were
my *Vogue* and *Elle* magazines (well, temporarily anyway). They
were replaced by my monthly baby mags – they were fantastic.
I highly recommend choosing one (just the one, mind you . . .
not the 10 that I used to purchase monthly . . . they all just
aren't necessary!) because they are brilliant at giving you
information on things like helping you decide on which
strollers or prams to buy, baby feeding issues, what to pack to
bring to the hospital, and a whole host of topics which always
seem to relate to what you are going through at that point.

But, of course, getting this sort of information from magazines and books (incidentally, I also have more than 30 books on pregnancy and birth with titles ranging from *Using Reflexology During Birth* to *Breathing Techniques During Labour* – see page 311 for a list of the ones I found most useful) is just not like the real thing. I wanted to hear a doctor on the other end of the phone for reassurance on all my worries.

I found myself constantly calling the office to ask them ridiculous questions which, at the time, seemed hugely important to me. Could I have egg-based mayonnaise in my sandwiches? What about pasteurized and non-pasteurized cheese? How come I was allowed Parmesan even though it was not pasteurized? Decaf or no coffee at all? Oh GOD – HELP! Every new thing worried me. I had been so concerned about actually getting pregnant and now a whole new set of worries had descended on me.

I would also call my doctor up to discuss the color of my vomit and to ask if it was hurting the baby! When I look back at this I realize I must have been such a pain in the bum but, at the time, I was paranoid that I might cause my baby harm. I also know from talking to other new mums that I am not the only pregnant woman to turn into a self-obsessed, neurotic, psychotic creature!

We soon realized, after seeing the amount of paraphernalia at my older sister Nathalie's house (she has three gorgeous little boys), that the amount of "stuff" required to care for just one offspring would mean that we would have to move out of our flat.

Easier said than done. We had only just moved in and Jamie was also in the midst of filming *Jamie's Kitchen* and setting up a new restaurant, so we had a lot on our plate. It was up to me to organize the move because, with everything else going on, it was too much for Jamie to even comprehend.

We were out driving one weekend when we spotted a lovely house for sale on the corner of a beautiful square in Hampstead. It just felt like "the one" and I knew instantly which room would be right for the nursery. So I set to thinking about how I was going to decorate it.

After much money wrangling and dealing it was ours. Now this really was our first proper home . . . more importantly, it had STAIRS! But it needed an awful lot of work and there would be no guarantee (especially from the contractors – surprise surprise) that we would be in before the baby was born. This was not how I had imagined it at all. We had six months to gut the house, damp-proof it, decorate it and get the nursery done (that was my main objective!).

THE JOYS OF MORNING SICKNESS

Now, enjoying the pregnancy is all very well until you discover the true meaning of MORNING SICKNESS. That was my first sign that being preggers can sometimes be quite yucky!

It makes me laugh to remember the chat I had with Nathalie. I was about seven weeks pregnant at the time and I confided that I felt very well and not sick at all. I was worried that perhaps something was wrong with my pregnancy or maybe I wasn't pregnant at all. Nat assured me that very soon

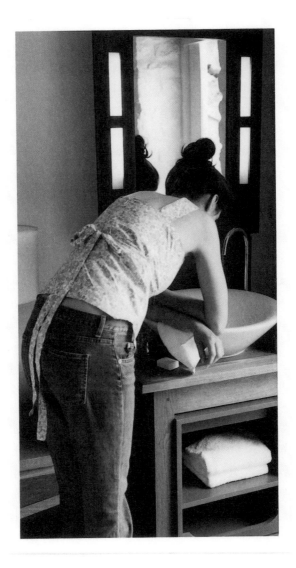

Thanks J for taking this
picture — nice memory! xxx

I might experience this morning sickness that all pregnant women talk about but not everyone goes through. There are the lucky few who sail through their pregnancy with no sickness or nausea at all. However, I was not to be one of them . . . typical!

Jamie was away in Australia at this time. I remember I woke very early one morning with a horrible, overwhelming sick feeling. One thing my mum had suggested just the night before was that to smell a cut lemon would help with nausea. Well, it may have worked for Mum, but no sooner had I crawled into bed with my lemon than I had to run to the bathroom and be sick. I was so shocked, as it all happened so quickly. The retching was horrendous and painful. It brought back memories of my childhood when I had whooping cough which made me sick so that I felt I couldn't breathe. I wasn't actually all that sick properly until a few weeks later on, but for now the intense and very tiring retching was to happen every morning for five months like clockwork. Weirdly, I would wake up feeling sick and hungry at the same time. I would retch first and then wolf food down straightaway. I have to admit that after the very first time I gave a little smile as I felt that things were now happening and I was really going to have a baby. But that smile soon faded after a couple of miserable mornings spent leaning over the sink . . .

We had still not told anyone about the baby as it was too early. Of course, my mum and both my sisters knew and we were dying to tell Jamie's family but we just wanted to wait those few weeks more before we announced it . . .
plus we wanted to tell Jamie's family when we were all together, but, as his schedule was so hectic, we had to wait.

It's always quite stressful being in the public eye and trying to keep a secret like that. I naively thought that as Jamie was the well-known one it would be him suffering all the hassle and pressure from the media and the paparazzi often waiting outside our house. But it seemed that ever since I discovered I was pregnant I was being asked by various newspaper journalists if I was expecting; and this was practically every time I left the house. I remember once, a journalist rang my doorbell incessantly, insisting that she knew I was pregnant. I don't know where journalists get their information from, but this time their sources were all pretty hot! The woman who rang the doorbell even produced a bunch of flowers congratulating me, which I thought was bizarre. I kept telling her over and over again that I wasn't pregnant. I didn't want to accept her flowers but she was insistent. It turned out that she was from the *Mirror* and they decided to run with the story anyway, even though we hadn't confirmed it.

It became such a pressure every time I left the house, as I had never really experienced the paparazzi before, especially on my own, and at times it was extremely intimidating. I felt I had a duty as a normal mum to keep my news private until the "safe" 12-week stage and then have the joy of telling all my close family and friends about our news rather than them finding out via a newspaper or magazine. But unfortunately that wasn't to be.

A couple of weeks before my 12-week sonogram, the story of our pregnancy was out. We had just been for a check-up at the hospital (I was having regular monitoring because of all the treatment I'd been through) very early in the morning, and after we'd dropped Jamie off at work I went home looking forward to a toasted banana sandwich with honey (and I mean that's really all I had thought about since I had woken up!). But no sooner had I closed my front door than the buzzer rang. I peeked through the intercom and there stood a journalist. Don't ask me how I knew he was one, I just did. It suddenly dawned on me that he wasn't alone – about five others were lurking around outside the house as well. It was crazy, ridiculous and – not to mention – embarrassing. What on earth would my neighbors think? I had never experienced this level of press attention before, not even with Jamie, and it was extremely unnerving. I tried to pretend that I wasn't in, which meant I had to crawl across the floor to shut the shutters and turn off all the lights. How silly was all this? It was bloody obvious that I was in – I needed to master the art of hiding out! I didn't even turn on my TV in case they could see the light from it through the shutters. They must have stayed out there for at least two hours. Talk about being desperate. When I finally emerged from my "prison" there was only one die-hard journalist left and I began to feel a bit sorry for him so I politely answered all his questions.

Suddenly I gave up trying to deny that I was expecting – it was too much of a struggle and had been in the *Mirror* anyway – so our very special and private news was out. The barrage of phone calls from close friends and family didn't stop. The sad thing is that the papers had managed to take away the excitement of breaking the news to them ourselves.

SO, WHAT WAS GOING ON INSIDE ME?

The weird and fascinating thing about the very early stages of pregnancy is that all these amazing things are going on inside your body, yet you cannot see the physical evidence straightaway. I remember reading in one of my many magazines that at around six weeks of pregnancy your fetus is the size of a rice grain and only a couple of weeks after that it was likened to the size of a baby broad bean – this always used to make Jamie and me laugh. Why did everything have to be compared to FOOD!

You really cannot stop thinking about the fact that you have a little living thing inside your tummy and the fact that you cannot feel it or see any evidence of it is just incredible. But the physical side to your pregnancy is thrust upon you sooner than I ever imagined it would be. The morning sickness was the first sign that I got but a lot of mums and friends have told me that their boobs were the first part of their body to change. They either became extremely sore or just two sizes bigger. Later on in my pregnancy, and also when I was breastfeeding, I used to make my friends laugh when I would run up the stairs holding on to my enlarged

boobs like they were prize watermelons – they were so
sensitive and painful. What a sight!

The next visible sign is probably your tummy. I certainly
noticed a change around the 10- or 11-week stage, when you
perhaps look a little full, but this of course all depends on
your body shape. I looked a bit bloated (you know, the sort
of bloated you get after a big meal!) up to about four and a
half months – so frustrating as I wanted my tummy
to start showing properly. But before long I was looking in
the mirror at a girl with a football shoved up her shirt!

Jamie wanted to be so involved at every stage of the
pregnancy, but there wasn't an awful lot he could do to help
at this point. Importantly, though, he fed me heaps of great
hearty food, like fish pie and soups full of fresh vegetables,
to keep my energy up and give me all the essential nutrients
which are necessary during this first trimester.

FOOD HABITS

Well, it's obviously funny for me to be writing about
anything to do with food, considering who my husband is,
but, contrary to popular belief, I am actually quite interested
in it. I like my food and, especially since having my girls,
I really enjoy cooking it as well. But, I have to admit that a
few years back, and especially when Jamie and I moved in
together for the first time, I was partial to the odd frozen
dinner or, dare I even say it, Pot Noodle (I can feel Jamie
cringing now). Due to the nature of his job, Jamie has always
worked nights so I have had to learn to fend for myself in the

kitchen. When we first moved to London I was modeling and would be exhausted after long shoot days so when I got back to the flat, the very thought of cooking something from scratch was inconceivable! But, of course, as time went on I started to learn a lot about food – well, I had no choice really!

When I became pregnant I decided to change my diet, as I am sure many women do when they realize that they are carrying a little human being inside them. It just makes sense. From that moment I have never eaten a frozen dinner again. Instead I got into making minestrone soup, one-pot stews – anything full of really tasty veg and I knew that all this was doing me good. It was also really easy to prepare.

FOOD CRAVINGS

Cravings are a classic and common sign of pregnancy, so I was quite looking forward to having some. You know the thing – you read about women or see them in films digging into pizza topped with anchovies and pineapple, or eating pickled gherkins slathered in custard, while decorating the nursery in paint-splattered overalls! When I did first get them it didn't surprise me, but I did think that they were a bit strange. Raw spaghetti dipped in Marmite as a little snack before dinner – well, pasta bows were a little hard on the teeth! I would advise anyone who has a similar craving to try the wholemeal spaghetti as it is much softer!

In my first trimester with Poppy I became obsessed with "old-school food" (for want of a better name). I am not sure how best to describe it, but I suddenly wanted to go back to basics; to have things like porridge or eggs – hearty, nourishing stuff. One particular morning after my usual bout of sickness, I had a very strong craving to eat an egg – but it had to be poached (any other way of preparing egg and I would have rushed to the bathroom again). The only trouble was, I had absolutely no idea how to make one. After trying to contact Jamie, Mum and my two sisters to no avail, I managed to get through to Nicky in Jamie's office. Now, I knew that she wouldn't have a clue either, so I asked her to call her mum to get the information for me! At last, after waiting a full hour in my pajamas, pan at the ready, I finally got to poach my egg . . . I devoured it in one go and loved it, and from that morning on, after my ten minutes of retching over the toilet, I would either call down to Jamie to get my poached egg going, or I'd have everything ready for when I went down to the kitchen. I had become an obsessed poached-egg-eating freak! And do you know what? Since those cravings, I've not eaten a poached egg (not even during my second pregnancy) and, quite frankly, I never really want to see one again as long as I live!

When it came to lunchtime, I developed a love of egg and watercress sandwiches – something I hadn't had since school. I loved having picnics in our local park and would take these little sandwiches with me (crusts cut off, naturally!) along with dips and slices of raw carrot and cucumber. I was crazy about snacks and I also loved anything salty. I would often take little packets of soy sauce to use as a dipping sauce for . . . well, anything! In fact, I could've drunk the soy sauce! Anchovies were also a big favorite of mine. I

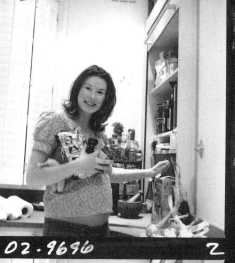
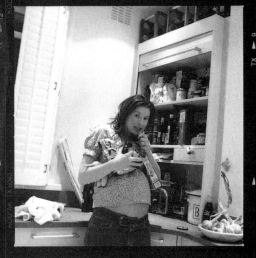
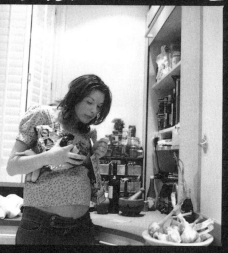

02·9696

2

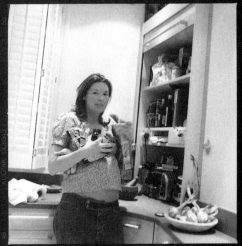
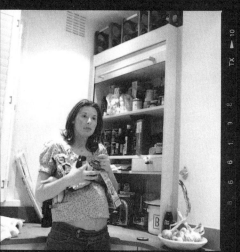
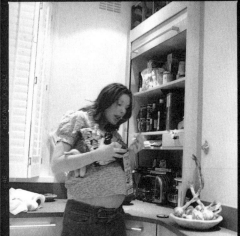

even cooked pasta for my picnics, putting it into Tupperware boxes with little individual packets of ketchup . . . oh YUCK, what was I thinking? Cold pasta with ketchup – what would Gordon Ramsay say?

It was all so bizarre (especially as I didn't have cravings the second time around with Daisy). My friend Lindsey, who was pregnant with Joel around the same time as I was with Daisy, had strong cravings for condensed milk and hot horseradish sauce. She would eat them straight out of the jar by the spoonful (although not mixed together!).

I also became a little partial to the odd afternoon tea with scones, jam and Earl Grey tea – oh, so civilized. Again, I didn't ever have these little obsessions with my second pregnancy, but perhaps that had more to do with the fact that I was running around after an adventurous crawling baby and didn't have time to fiddle around whipping up cream for my scones!

I loved fish and chips. Jamie used to treat me on Saturday lunchtimes when he wasn't working, by driving me to Golbourne Road Fish Shop, where they do the best fish and chips in London. They serve them in a little cardboard lunch box with a wedge of lemon (Jamie always had a big pickled chilli on the side of his). They were so delicious. We would even drive to a picturesque spot – the Golbourne Housing Estate! – where we would have to duck down in the car in case any of the kids on their bikes banged on the window and asked Jamie if he could cook for them. Well, we couldn't drive any farther as it was essential that the fish and chips were piping hot. Jamie was more concerned that the batter would go soggy, whereas I was just starving! So, that for me was my ultimate treat when I was pregnant. Fortunately, now my hormone levels are back to normal, I see a treat as dinner out at a nice restaurant (thank you very much, Jamie, in case you are reading this!).

OTHER ODDITIES

It wasn't just my taste buds going haywire. It seemed that pregnancy heightened my sense of smell. Everything had to smell "fresh" to me – that's the only way I can describe it. But, ironically, I didn't like air fresheners – oh, it's a barmy old world! We had only just recently moved into our flat and it had been freshly decorated. The smell of paint had a really peculiar effect and became quite distressing to me. I hated it. I only had to come in after being out all day to be hit by the powerful paint smell and would instantly want to throw up. It was so frustrating. I tried to counteract the smell with lots of those plug-in air fresheners in every room, but they really got to me as well.

Perhaps the strangest craving, though, was my obsession with rubber . . . not in a kinky way, unfortunately for Jamie! I became completely addicted to the smell and this happened with both my pregnancies. I loved the taste and smell of it and, most weirdly of all, I loved chewing it (but not actually eating it – I drew the line at that!). I would chew for hours on anything rubbery – be it a pencil case that I found at my mum's house in my old room, the handles of screwdrivers, and, in my second pregnancy, even Poppy's little rubber

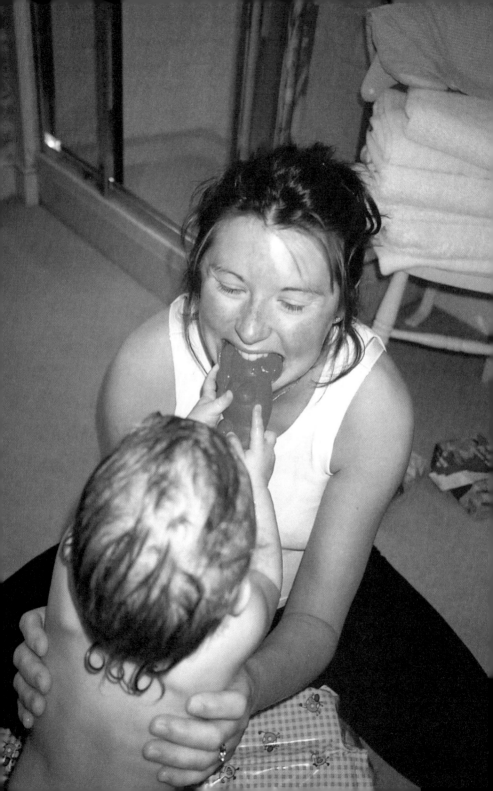

ducks and toys that she played with in the bath. We used
to fight over them when we bathed together! If I found I had
a free 10 minutes I would dash down to our local hardware
store in Hampstead and linger around the section that was
filled with rubber-ended hammers and screwdrivers, rubber
piping, etc. . . . It smelled divine to me! Obviously I had to
keep a low profile when doing this, so subtlety was the key
and I always had to buy something once I was in there for
fear of being arrested for lurking. That shop made quite a
tidy profit from my pregnancy craving! I don't have a rational
explanation for this very strange behavior, but as soon as
I had had the babies it disappeared and I have never felt
the need to do it since – THANK GOD!

TIME FOR MATERNITY WEAR YET?

I was really looking forward to wearing maternity clothes,
but I realize now that it wasn't the prospect of actually
wearing them that appealed, but more the idea that I could
be big enough to change my wardrobe so drastically. It was
just another exciting aspect of being pregnant and getting
bigger. Little did I know that the clothes themselves weren't
quite so exciting.

It's hard to know when to start buying larger clothes. I tried
to get away with it until I reached about three and a half
months when I found that my precious jeans were no longer
buttoning up. Having had a quick look at some of the shops
which sold maternity clothes, I felt crestfallen because there
was really nothing I liked. Everything looked old-fashioned –

no matter how hard the shops tried to make them seem young and different, they just screamed BORING PREGNANCY CLOTHES! However, the one excellent thing that these clothes do have going for them is that they are designed for comfort which, in the end, is the most important thing.

I felt that I would take the other clothes option of upping my size bit by bit, especially with my jeans. I went from a size 8 to a size 14 in a matter of months. It was hilarious! I have always been very thin. I was the girl in the playground who the others teased, shouting things like "there goes beanpole – careful or you might fall down a drain." So, inevitably, when I became pregnant I was ready for the "look it's a toothpick that swallowed a beach ball" teases! I was actually very pleased when I started to blossom and the toothpick turned into a chopstick with a beach ball tum and a rugby ball bum!

Anyway, when it came to shopping for bigger-sized "normal" clothes, I found the trouble with moving up a size was that I would be fine for a few months but then I would have to do another batch of shopping to accommodate for the next stage of sizing. I did manage to find some real die-hard clothes that seemed to last my whole pregnancy though. One thing was a really lovely soft high-neck sweater with a tie detail at the waist. It wasn't actual maternity wear, but it seemed to stretch with me and it was so comfy. The other favorite was a pair of jeans. Now, after buying countless cheap jeans to try and see me through (which were okay but they never seemed to fit properly on the bum, hence many a paparazzi picture of my plumber butt hanging out with my

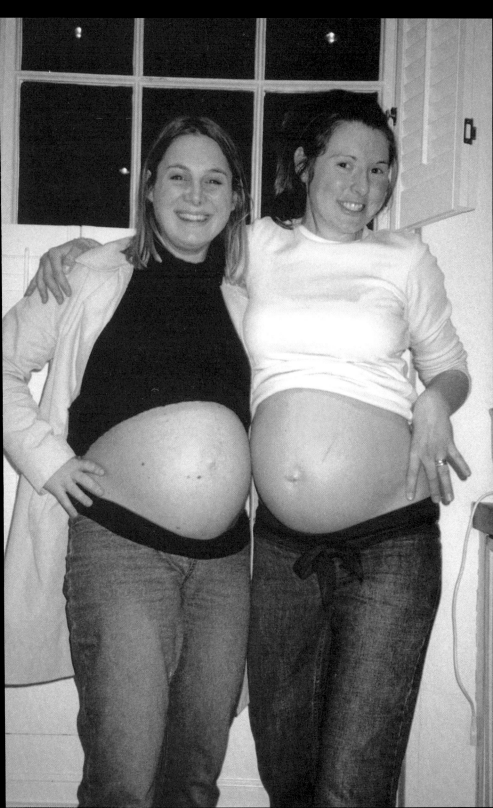

belly stretched the other way to even up the balance!) I came across a brilliant pair which I had seen advertised in a baby magazine. They were made by Juicy Couture and were pricey, but they lasted me all the way through my pregnancy and beyond. Essentially, they were maternity jeans which were designed to fit under the bump (which I preferred); they also fit really well over the bum and with a straight leg they fit my shape perfectly. They even had a subtle elastic-waist panel (like all other maternity jeans out there) but it wasn't wide, so I didn't feel like I was being strapped together by a bandage. I really loved wearing them and I hope that they will see me through – God willing – any future pregnancies!

The clothes you wear during your last few months are obviously dictated by which season your baby is due. For both of my girls I was noticeably showing all the way through the winter, so I was able to cover myself up, but I longed to be showing off my bumps in pretty summer dresses and cotton tops. I felt sure it would be easier to dress a big tum in summer attire as opposed to covering it up in warm winter sweaters and overcoats and looking twice the size!

Oh God, now I think back, there was MANY an outfit worn by me that was hideous and very unflattering. Unfortunately, I could not just put it down to a bad mistake and forget about it. My outfit choices seemed to be endlessly documented in ridiculous celebrity magazines as the "celeb mum – how not to dress" look. That will teach me to wear Jamie's red and blue T-shirt with some silly slogan written across it, with his tracksuit bottoms and his horrible smelly anorak that has a fur trim!

I looked shocking. But to be fair, I was two days away from my due date and was moving to a new house. The pressure was on and I was not about to start worrying about trivial things like winning the "best-dressed celeb mum" award at a time like that. (But just so you know, I do still look back at that picture and cringe!)

I have a friend Jadene who has two gorgeous little boys. When she was pregnant with her first, her fashion sense went right out the window. She used to make me laugh so much with her stories. Once she had been invited to a Michael Jackson concert when she was about eight months pregnant. She was desperate to get out and have a good time as it meant she could dress up and feel fabulous for once! After many frustrating hours in front of her wardrobe, trying to squeeze into her size-10 trousers and sexy tops, it just wasn't happening. So in a moment of hormonal hedonism she opted for her leopard-print silky catsuit and black high heels. Her excuse was that it was "comfortable" (well, I'm sure it was but there is a reason why maternity wear shops DO NOT stock leopard-print catsuits – or any catsuits for that matter!). Of course the looks on her friends' faces as she arrived at the concert were a picture, although I did forget to mention that she is an extremely beautiful model who is 5'11" with gorgeous tumbling blonde hair, so I'm sure she would have looked fab in a sack! As she recalled this story to me many months later, I couldn't help but think, "What the hell was she doing with a leopard print catsuit in her wardrobe anyway?"

I had always thought that maternity wear and evenings out were not synonymous with each other but after hearing Jadene's catsuit story I was convinced! When I was pregnant (and showing) I had the odd dress or two that saw me through the very few nights that I did venture out on the town. One was a black jersey knee-length dress with a ribbon-tie detail and a low V-neck front which I wore to my surprise 27th birthday at a restaurant in Birmingham (after the Good Food Show one needs a decent surprise or two as I've spent every birthday for the last five years there – arrrrrgh!). With the dress I wore some simple low heels and fishnet tights and I thought I looked pretty good for a six-months preggers girl! But I couldn't wear it out to every occasion so I often found myself standing in front of my wardrobe glassy-eyed and disappointed after trying to squeeze into summer dresses, hoping they would look cute over maternity jeans and heels . . . well, if it worked for Kate Moss it could work for me, couldn't it? Obviously not! So I either said no to invites out, unless it was to a friend's house for a night in with the girls and an array of Cadbury's chocolate bars, or I wore my little black dress again!

When I was pregnant the second time, I decided to try a little harder when it came to maternity fashion. With a possible invite to the London Restaurant Awards and being eight months pregnant it was time to get sorted. After weeks of trying on dress after dress I finally found a gorgeous knee-length one with thick straps and a bit of a twist detail on the

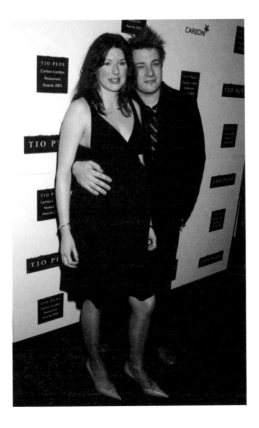

boob area . . . black again but it just seemed to work. I think Cat
Deeley wore the same one when she presented an episode of
Fame Academy but it looked a damn sight more gorgeous on
her I have to admit! All dressed up with chandelier earrings
and turquoise high heels I thought I scrubbed up pretty well.
But, rather unfortunately, I was photographed and in the
Evening Standard the next day I just looked puffy and round!

Looking back now, I don't think it really matters what you
wear when you're pregnant, whether you're going down to the

shops or out for dinner, because you will be blooming and glowing and that is what people will see. I know that Jamie found me unbelievably attractive when I was pregnant – so when I look back at these pictures of me looking like a blob I laugh first but then I realize that inside me was one of our gorgeous girls. That alone makes me think I looked stunning.

Consequently, I wore that dress just the other night but over my jeans with a big wide belt and my trusty cowboy boots (à la my style guru, Sienna Miller!) and I felt pretty good in it. So if you do buy maternity wear for going out in, have a look to see if you can come up with some new outfits after the baby is born – better than having them put away at the back of the wardrobe.

UNDERWEAR ISSUES

Another major issue was underwear. Bras were definitely more of a problem than maternity clothes. It became an ongoing nightmare and even now the problem hasn't gone away!

First, underwear is extremely important when you are pregnant, especially if you want to avoid the saggy-boobies syndrome! I had always been a 34B ever since I can remember, but in the last three years I have seen my boobs go from a 34B to a 38D then back down . . . way, way down . . . to a 34A, then back up again in full effect for Daisy's pregnancy then down again. Up, down, up, down – no wonder my underwear drawer resembles a bargain bin!

Basically, I was not prepared for the size increase and the amount of time that I was going to have to spend trying on maternity bras that didn't seem to fit me for very long! Well, my only advice on this is to GET FITTED PROPERLY BY A TRAINED BRA FITTER as I call them, but basically any of the lovely ladies in the lingerie sections of large department stores. I found they were fantastic in terms of helpful and knowledgeable assistance and there was a great selection of underwear and it was good value for money. However, I did spend a lot of time looking through catalogues as well, hoping that it might be the solution to picking the right size. I didn't realize that there were so many choices – you have night-feeding bras, day-feeding bras, sporty-looking bras, leopard-print bras. So confusing! In the end I decided to opt for the sporty-looking bra as it could double up as a nighttime feeding one as well and it just looked so comfortable.

The next issue facing me was to choose the right size. In the catalogues it said "opt for the size that you usually wore before you were pregnant, e.g., 34 or 36," so I opted for the 34 and hoped for the best. But not one to do things by halves, I chose two in every color as I was convinced that these were the ones to be wearing. When they finally arrived none of them fitted properly and they certainly didn't look as nice on me as they did on the pregnant model in the catalogue photograph! I have to laugh when I open the bottom drawer in the nursery to see a pile of maternity and breastfeeding bras in every color – all nice and pristine awaiting an outing! So it's probably best to get measured properly every few weeks and buy from a department store.

With my second pregnancy, the midwife told me that the best thing to do is to wait until two weeks before your due date and then go and have a professional bra fitting. The reason

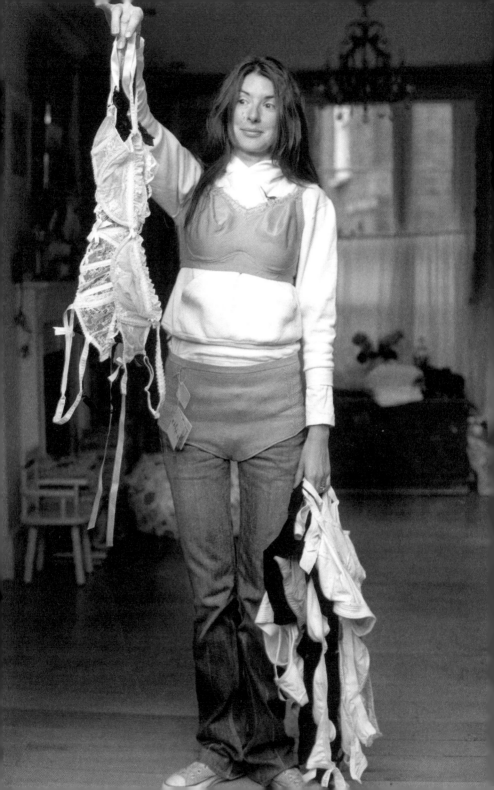

it's good to wait until this time is that this is when you'll do the most growing as your milk is preparing to come in.

I remember once, for some reason (although, bless him for doing it), Jamie was trying to cheer me up after I had spent the millionth morning hunched over the toilet retching for dear life. He decided on a quick trip to Selfridges to treat me (although I think this had some benefit to him!) to some very gorgeous and sexy underwear. Little did he know that sexy underwear was not on the top of my list of treats at that point – a two-hour foot massage, followed by countless girls' magazines and a large bar of chocolate would have been more like it, but who am I to complain? A few hours later he came home laden with shopping bags galore, full of beautiful matching underwear, apart from the odd thong thrown in there! But, of course, not one of the pieces fit me – the panties were too tight, the bras were too small and underwired and don't even mention the thongs! He begged me to keep them for when I wasn't pregnant but, to this day, they are still all beautifully wrapped in tissue paper in my chest of drawers waiting for me to fit into them. Funnily enough, I tried a few on yesterday and, typically, they are too big. I don't know whether to laugh or cry! I suppose the moral of that story is don't waste lots of money on fancy underwear when your boobs are increasing in size so quickly. Save it until after the baby, then it really will be a treat, if you've got the time or the energy!

CHAPTER THREE

The Second Trimester

SCANS AND DIARIES

This part of your pregnancy is often referred to as the best time – when your hormones have settled down a bit and you don't feel so tired. My appetite started to come back in full force, although I was still suffering from morning sickness. It would make Jamie laugh, as every morning when I woke up I couldn't even talk about food or look at a commercial on TV without rushing to the bathroom to stick my head down the toilet, but as soon as I had actually been sick I would discuss with him in great detail what I was going to have for breakfast – ironically it was my favorite meal of the day.

At the same time, I began to intensely dislike the sight, smell and taste of tea or coffee (so my afternoon tea and scone was out the window). I've heard that this is really common with pregnant women, but it doesn't cease to amaze me that one morning you can love something and the next minute you can't stand it.

But this trimester is a really exciting time as well, as this is when you start to really see that something is happening to your body – your boobs are definitely getting bigger, your trousers become tighter, you might be feeling bloated, but your sickness may stop (hurray!). It's also the time when you start to have appointments and check-ups.

The first appointment with your hospital or doctor is

always so exciting. Usually you don't get to visit the doctor until you're three months pregnant, which is when you have the 12-week scan. This is the first time that you will see your little baby and it is so exciting! However, because of the fertility treatment I'd been receiving, I had been seeing my doctor for checks and early scans from when I was about four weeks pregnant. So I was lucky enough to see my little Poppy's heartbeat at this point. Usually at these scans you are able to take away pictures – I 'm lucky enough to have one of these early ones of Poppy which is just amazing.

At this stage of my pregnancy Jamie was away a lot working, so we hardly saw each other, which was difficult. Because so many exciting things were happening, or about to happen, he would get lengthy phone calls from me describing in detail every little thing about the baby and how I was feeling. I didn't let him get a word in edgeways!

I spent a lot of time at home with my mum when Jamie was away, as I felt safe there and I knew that she would look after me the best! On the odd occasion, though, especially in my first trimester, I would surprise Jamie by hiding in his hotel when he was off around the country on his book tour, so that when he came back after a book signing in some lonely city I would be waiting in the room. I used to get very excited, as I knew that he would never expect me to be so spontaneous. On one such occasion I was staying at my mum's and I hatched a plan to catch a train to one of Jamie's hotels. He had begged me to come along on the whole tour, but I was still feeling so dreadful in the mornings, I told him it wouldn't be possible. . . . I was a good actress! When

I arrived at the hotel I told the staff that it was a surprise, then found myself an appropriate hiding place in his room (they must have thought I was mad!). Well, he was thoroughly surprised – I think he thought that I was part of the furniture as he walked straight past me, but then he did a double take and was totally shocked. I vowed to try and surprise him at least once on each trip.

Now, having said that, there was no way I was going to surprise him on his month-long tour around Australia (although I have a massive fondness for the place) because I am so very terrified of flying. Having done the trip once before, unless I could be knocked out like Mr. T from *The A Team*, I wasn't going to be surprising anyone!

His going away couldn't have been more terribly planned. As I just said, all the exciting things that come along with the second trimester were about to start happening, although I'm sure he didn't miss the raucous retching that could be heard from our bedroom at 6:00 am EVERY morning (for five months!).

I remember the afternoon he left. We spent our last hours together trying to set up our new camera phones so that we would be able to send pictures to each other while he was away. We took all these pictures of my bump at various angles so Jamie could look at it when he missed Poppy (although at the time we didn't name the bump Poppy, as we had our hearts set on a boy's name, but I won't mention that as you never know, one day ...). Anyway, subsequently my camera phone was unable to send images overseas – typical – but in the end I think it worked out better, as when I went to meet him at the airport he was completely surprised. He couldn't believe how big my bump had grown and it's all he talked about on the way home, so it was worth it just for that.

Anyway, with all this traveling that he was doing, it was impossible to book hospital appointments around his schedule. It used to really make me laugh as Nicola tried to sort the appointments out with me. If I told her that I had a 12-week scan that had to be around a certain date she used to check his diary and get back to me saying, "Well, perhaps he can take 45 minutes off around November 30 – can they hold on till then?" That would have made me almost six blinkin' months pregnant!

When you're pregnant for the first time, you do tend to become immersed in your own world of "babies babies babies" and dates, trimesters, weeks, months, due dates and scans; so much so that you expect everyone around you to understand the great importance of it all. I don't think Nix had a clue about trimesters or scans – I must have been such a boring friend at that time! In the end I decided to ask the doctor's secretary if she could liaise with Nicky to sort the dates out, as it all just became too confusing! Mind you, I should have foreseen this particular problem arising. Here's a story for you . . .

When we got married, we were to have a wedding rehearsal in the church. I was really excited about it, naturally, and it was all planned and organized. But then a Sainsbury's commercial had to be booked into Jamie's diary urgently a couple of days before and there was NO getting out of it. It meant that he couldn't make the wedding rehearsal, which I was furious about, to say the least. Seeing that I was obviously distressed, it was laughably suggested that I bring the wedding party up to the supermarket and perhaps we could conduct it there. What? Down the meat or fish aisle? I don't think so! The only aisle I wanted to walk down was the church aisle, which I did, but in the rehearsal I didn't marry Jamie – I married his best friend, Andy the Gasman! At least someone knew what they were doing come our wedding day, and I won't let Jamie forget about it either!

Anyway, back to the matters of scanning and diaries. We finally established a date for my 12-week scan and I was told it would also involve having a nuchal scan which measures the fold of skin at the back of the baby's neck (to assess the risk of possible heart defects or Down syndrome – I've explained more in the glossary of terms at the end of the book). We asked if they could very kindly keep the clinic open late, as Jamie was filming *Jamie's Kitchen* at the time in our house (so if anyone wonders why, during that show, I was, let's say . . . short-tempered, hopefully this book gives a little insight into the reasons why!). There was so much anticipation and excitement that we were going to see our baby properly for the first time. I just can't describe how I was feeling. On the other hand, I was incredibly nervous that the technician would turn on the screen and then tell me it was all a mistake and that I wasn't pregnant at all. I needed complete reassurance at that stage and could easily have moved into the hospital on a permanent basis and married the technician!

Now, after all that – and keep in mind that I had drunk my

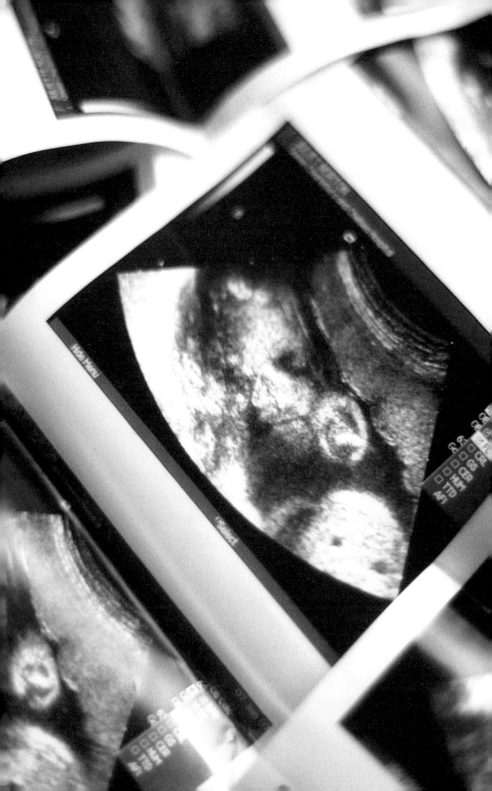

two liters of water (although just a liter would have done, as this helps to make the scan clearer) – I was just that little bit too early to have the nuchal scan, since they couldn't get a complete and accurate reading. Nonetheless, that experience with Jamie and our baby was utterly amazing.

OW! THE BABY'S KICKING!

Now possibly THE MOST exciting thing to happen during your pregnancy is feeling the baby kick for the first time, and from then onward until it is born.

I was fascinated about this, way before I became pregnant. My first experience of seeing a baby kick in its mum's tummy was when my sister Nat, who was about eight months pregnant with her first son, Jake, was sitting in my mum's kitchen. Suddenly this hand-shaped thing pushed against her tummy. It was so quick, yet I couldn't forget about it. I didn't realize that this was what happened – it was fascinating. It really was the identical shape to his little hand. I couldn't wait for the same thing to happen to me.

Of course, while you are pregnant, you often spend many hours daydreaming about what the hell is going on inside you. When I first found out I was pregnant, for example, after peeing on the magic stick, I ran down the stairs, put on my Destiny's Child CD and jigged around to "Survivor" but then suddenly became aware that inside me there was a tiny, tiny rice grain who was probably trying to catch 40 winks, and here I was dancing around like a lunatic! After reading all the pregnancy books and mags that I could get my hands on, I was then counting down the days until my baby started to kick.

I used to imagine the feeling would be like a real hard kick that would wind me, but my mum said that us three girlies (Nat, Lisa and me) all felt like little butterflies in her tummy at the beginning, so I waited to have these feelings myself.

I remember vividly when I felt the first little movement. I was lying on our sofa chatting on the phone to Jamie's mum when suddenly I felt a little pop in my tummy, very low down. It felt like a bubble bursting and I instinctively knew it was our baby and not just a bit of gas. It was so exciting! I didn't move a muscle in case she was going to do it again. I waited and waited but nothing happened. She was obviously giving me just a little taste of what was to come! I immediately called Jamie, who was in Australia on his month-long tour. He was disappointed that he was not there to witness the first time Poppy bubbled in my tum, but she soon made up for that. A few months later, our main entertainment at night was watching her dance around in my belly on a regular basis.

Poppy was a real kicker and, for some reason, if I drank a glass of Coke it really got her going. She would jump around inside me like a kangaroo. When I was pregnant with Daisy, I felt her kick very early on (at about 14 weeks), but she was generally a much calmer baby and would hardly ever move around. Although if I lay on my right side she would kick out like a little David Beckham! It's amazing just how different the two little babies were, even that early on.

I remember once reading an article that Jamie had written for a magazine where he described the joy of feeling Poppy move around in my tummy. I loved it when he said that when I was asleep he used to cuddle me from behind and hold my tummy, waiting for the baby to make a move. I suppose it was a little private moment for just the two of them. Sometimes you really forget about your partner when you are pregnant. I used to get so wrapped up in me and the baby that I would forget that Jamie was also part of this amazing experience. Reading that article gave me the insight that he was as fascinated and excited as I was.

IS THE BABY OKAY?

Once you establish that your baby is healthy and kicking like a trouper, I think one of the most common worries as you progress further into your pregnancy is whether your baby is okay when it's not kicking or whether it is kicking enough. I naturally worried about ALL of these things ALL of the time.

If I was really busy during the day I didn't notice whether the baby was kicking or not. What I did come to realize was that while I was active during the day, she was asleep and while I was asleep at night, she would be her most active. Only slightly comforted by this thought, Jamie and I decided to buy a machine that would allow us to monitor the baby's heartbeat ourselves. There are actually lots of these available at quite reasonable prices – particularly from shops like Target, or mother-and-baby catalogues. They look a bit like CD players with headphones. You can strap them to your tummy and listen to your baby's heartbeat through the headphones, as if you are listening to music – how fantastic!

Jamie and I were out shopping one day and we passed an excellent medical-supply shop just off Oxford Street. Weirdly, I'm interested in anything remotely medical or clinical, so I begged Jamie to go inside with me to have a look. It was the sort of shop that supplies to big hospitals, and so it had every kind of implement you could imagine! After much probing (from me, naturally) I was convinced by the medical expert behind the counter that we should buy the professional heartbeat monitor called a Doppler. It's the same one that is used in doctors' offices and hospitals and it came with a mini tube of gel. You smear this on your tummy and then move the monitor around just like a professional scan. Jamie literally had to drag me out of there when the shop assistant asked if I was interested in buying a mini sonogram machine . . . !

We couldn't wait to use the monitor when we got home. Typically, I could listen for hours to Poppy's heart, but after a while, Jamie would find other more juvenile uses for my precious equipment like checking his own heartbeat then telling me that I didn't have one as he couldn't find it! But at least we were all happy.

As good as it was to use the monitor, these constant checks could become a little too much, especially on those days when the baby was lying in a curled up position and it was hard to detect a heartbeat. This would send me into a wild panic and have me calling Jamie at work and making him stay on the line until we could hear it again. With our second baby, Daisy, the monitor became my most treasured piece of equipment. Whenever I had a bleed or similar scare I would rush for the Doppler just so I could hear her heartbeat. I found it incredibly reassuring.

MANY SLEEPING ISSUES

Now, along with all the amazing and wonderful aspects of pregnancy, you have to deal with the not-so-nice things as well. I've already mentioned the morning sickness (which, for me, was possibly the worst aspect of pregnancy) but, believe me, there are many, many others!

When I reached about 12 weeks, just going into my second trimester, I suddenly started to notice that I was having difficulty in getting to sleep and then actually having any sleep at all.

The first interruption was my constant need to pee. This had me getting up at least twice a night, which I found so hard to get used to. I've always been the sort of person who would never get up to go to the bathroom in the middle of the night – I would rather hold it in until morning. But when I was pregnant that wasn't an option. This started to get on my nerves after a while, especially as you read in countless nutrition and baby books you need to drink plenty of water. It would take me all day, right through to bedtime, to get through two liters (the recommended amount) so I had no choice – you can't win! It was always hard to get back to sleep after one of my regular visits to the bathroom, so every morning I felt exhausted.

Another of my common sleep interruptions was what I called "agitated legs." There is no other way to describe the feeling. Often I would sink into bed, looking forward to what might be a restful night, only to get this feeling of dead legs – almost like they were overtired and needed to be constantly moved and rubbed. I just couldn't keep them still and this could last for hours until I finally fell asleep. I haven't had it since the girls were born, but in both my pregnancies this occurred. So frustrating!

And yet another thing to deprive me of my sleep was one perhaps only akin to myself . . . my husband. When I was expecting (and this was with both girls), I liked to get into a lovely fresh bed with crisp sheets and I would lie there, the duvet tucked around me nice and tidy, with the pillow in just the right position. Sleeping in this organized fashion allowed me to at least cope with all the agitation I felt throughout the night. But, oh no, Jamie couldn't possibly manage to keep the bed, just slightly straight and tidy. I would always be the first one in bed as Jamie is a bit of a night worker (having said that, he is a bit of a day one too).

I would have finally drifted off to sleep when Jamie would get into bed and crash down on to the mattress, pulling the duvet across his side of the bed. He'd then chuck any excess pillows across the room. Now, I'm a bit like Monica from *Friends,* as you've probably noticed by now! I can't stand mess around me, and that goes for when I'm in bed too. This meant that I would have to get up, pick up the pillows, invariably have to pick up all his clothes which he had shed around the room and then straighten all the bed covers. (I know I am beginning to sound like the scary husband from the Julia Roberts film *Sleeping with the Enemy,* but that's pregnancy for you, and I suppose that's MEN for you too!)

This sleep deprivation carried on throughout my pregnancy. I was constantly irritated from the moment I went to sleep to the moment I woke up. I remember I used to say to Jamie (actually, I would usually wake him up to tell him – well, there's nothing worse than a contented, happily sleeping partner when you are wide awake and frustrated!) that I wouldn't mind if I was getting up in the middle of the night for a purpose, like feeding our little baby. I felt it would be so wonderful to comfort a crying baby. . . . Stop right there! How wrong I was. Little did I know that I'd be longing for those constant pee breaks instead!

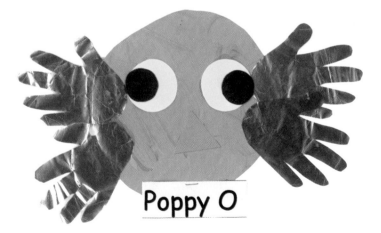

CHAPTER FOUR

The Third Trimester

LEAKY BOOBS . . .

Now apparently at this stage of your pregnancy you are meant
to feel full of beans and have the energy of a sprinter. . . . I am
not sure who made that load of garbage up, but for me it
wasn't the case at all. Although I can say that about three
weeks before my due date I had a sudden burst of energy that
I channeled into cleaning the house! This happened with
both pregnancies, and is a subject which I will touch upon
later in this chapter, as it often had very funny consequences!

When I was six months gone I began to feel properly
pregnant. I really started to show and I found it so exciting.
I remember waiting eagerly for my belly button to pop out
as it can sometimes do when you are about seven months
along. It reminded me of a little oven timer – one minute it
was an inny and the next, *ping*, and it was an outie.
Fascinating! (Dear God, what had happened to my social life?)

Another thing which really took me by surprise was – how
can I put it? – leaky boobs! This started when I was around
six months pregnant. On waking in the morning, I started to
notice that I had little dried patches circling my boobs. They
were slightly yellow in color – sounds disgusting doesn't it?
At first I panicked as I wondered if I had some sort of

infection. In my naivete I just couldn't work out what these patches were (a bit like crop circles!). Anyway, after a quick phone call to the fount of all knowledge – my mum – she assured me that it was probably the onset of my colostrum. This is the very thin watery milk that precedes the full-fat stuff later on. I wanted to catch this colostrum at work – this really was fascinating (way better than my distant social life!) – but it mostly happened at night when I was asleep.

When I was washing up one night after a delicious dinner that *I* had cooked for us, Jamie made a comment about the lack of seasoning in the minestrone. Now, at any other time this comment would have been laughed off with a very sharp retort, but on this pregnant occasion I didn't feel in the mood for witty repartee, so . . . I cried and I shouted, and as I did (much to Jamie's shock) my boobs started to leak through my top! Talk about a great bodily tactic to stop an argument in its tracks! As I lifted up my top we both looked in amazement as my boobs released this watery colostrum right before our eyes in little steady flows from each nipple. So at last we had managed to watch it in action. It's a shame really that we don't have colostrum all the time as never again during an argument have I been able to perform the same trick. It really was an excellent diversionary tool, especially if, like me, you had also scraped the side of your husband's prized car the same day!

From this point on I started to stock up on breast pads as I was fed up with having little incidents like my friends telling me to leave the dance floor immediately as I had two very visible damp circles on my shirt. Very attractive!

HEARTBURN

It was also around the seventh month of pregnancy that I discovered the real pain of heartburn. I had never understood what all the fuss was about when people said that they suffered from incredibly painful heartburn – until I was inflicted with it nearly every night for the last two months of both my pregnancies.

I wasn't sure what the main triggers were for it, but certainly if Jamie had cooked one of his very chilli- and spice-enriched dinners that would always be the culprit. Many a night I would wake up with a feeling of rising fire from my chest to my throat. I would prop myself up against my pillows, banging on my chest like a bloody gorilla trying to ease the acidic feeling. I would be so loud and fidgety that I used to end up downstairs sleeping on the sofa. So, I tried to eat slightly earlier than Jamie in the evening to avoid the food lying heavily on my tummy while I slept. This worked well, but it wasn't always enough. I was reluctant to use anything medical to help, though, as I was worried it would affect the baby. After many weeks of this I decided to give in and take a remedy. As my sister had been through the same thing with her pregnancies, she suggested that I try Gaviscon – a favorite of hers. On one particularly rough night it worked and I was able to eventually fall asleep after a lot of chest banging à la Tarzan! I was not partial to the liquid variety of Gaviscon though, and soon discovered that the more chalky pill form was for me. No longer was there an elegant candle and a good book on my bedside table –

instead, propped up against my lamp were three packs of lemon-flavored Gaviscon, a vaporizer which emitted a lemon smell (to help ward off morning sickness) and a packet of Breathe Right strips . . . yes, these helped me cure another of my nightly afflictions – how romantic!

It seems that I was not the only one to suffer from breathing problems in the third trimester. Many of my other pregnant friends also complained of the same problem, and mostly at night. For four months I had a continually blocked nose which would thrust itself upon me in the dead of night, every night. After telling my doctor about this he explained that an increase in progesterone causes the nasal lining to swell and partially block the airway, so it all became clear (but not my nose!).

I rooted around all the pharmacists to try and find an efficient, safe remedy to unblock my nasal passages. The most recommended thing was a product called Breathe Right – little sticky strips like bandages which you place across the bridge of your nose to help open up the nasal passages. They are like the sort of thing that you sometimes see athletes or race-car drivers wearing. The first night I used them – in fact, the second I put them on – I instantly noticed a difference. My whole nose seemed to clear and my nostrils felt fresh and open for the first time in ages. I would put these on every night as part of my bedtime routine – next it will be the false teeth and the leg bandages . . . poor Jamie!

After reading that section out loud to Jamie recently, he laughed his head off remembering all my bedtime paraphernalia. He also couldn't believe that I had had to endure such nightmarish nights. I don't think he was even aware that I was suffering from all these agitations on a nightly basis. Typical male!

I was fascinated at this stage to imagine what the baby looked like and how much it had grown – at around eight months your baby is about the size of a small watermelon. I would spend hours leafing through my pregnancy books checking out what my baby could do at this stage. I loved it when I read such lines as "your baby is able to suck his thumb now." It gave me great images to daydream about. Many of the pregnancy books I had were laid out in stages – either in trimesters or weeks. I liked the weekly guides best as it was easy to keep tabs on where I was during the pregnancy and I would look forward to checking my progress. Naturally, whether I wanted to or not, I don't think I ever picked up a pregnancy book when I was having my second baby because my first baby wouldn't allow it!

I find it so funny that most pregnant women will spend hours poring over books and watching television programs about pregnancy and birth ... and yet I don't know many friends who ever read past the labor and birth chapter about "your first weeks with your new baby!" I felt like I spent nine months trying to keep my babies safe and secure inside me, but then completely forgot that sooner or later they would be making their way out and then there would be a whole new set of things to worry about! I was completely focused on the here and now. I think that so much emphasis is put on the nine months of pregnancy that it's easy to forget you will then have this little person for the rest of your lives ...

So, help is what we needed. In Britain at around seven to

eight months of pregnancy you are given the opportunity to join your local prenatal class, to help you prepare for the birth and beyond. In certain areas you will be offered a chance to go to your local NHS classes, or you can pay to go to the NCT (National Childbirth Trust) classes. The two classes do vary slightly in content and what they teach you. The NCT classes focus more on the actual birth and delivery, including ways in which to deal and cope with it all, but they barely touch upon actually caring for your baby. Whereas the NHS classes focus more on the aftercare of you and the baby, as well as aspects of childcare straight after the birth (changing diapers, how to bathe your baby, etc). Both classes are equally helpful and a great thing to take part in during the last few weeks of pregnancy in the lead-up to your labor. We felt it was a really nice way to round off the whole experience.

Jamie and I decided to opt for our local NCT prenatal classes. I found out about them from the back of one of my countless magazines in a section entitled The National Childbirth Trust. If you call the number for their main headquarters, stating where you live, they will tell you where the closest NCT center is. Unlike the free NHS classes, you are normally asked to pay a fee of about £100 for the whole course; for that you get six two-hour classes with cookies and a cup of tea thrown in!

Coordinating Jamie's schedule was another nightmare for Nicky to organize. If she wasn't organizing his calender to fit around my fertile days, she was trying to arrange it around the prenatal classes. This was never in the job description when she applied – mind you, neither was dealing with my constant hormonal moods, like when she once dared to tell me that Jamie might possibly have to work on one of the NCT nights. (Poor girl, thank goodness she was my best friend – sorry, Nix!)

Of course, like all first-time parents, we had absolutely no idea what these classes were going to be like or, for that matter, what the people would be like who were attending them. Nevertheless, I was really excited and nervous on the day of our first class. I only wished that Jamie mirrored my boundless enthusiasm! He was absolutely dreading going. He was sure that it was just a women's thing and was paranoid that we would turn up and find that he was the only guy there surrounded by 15 heavily pregnant women! But, of course, it wasn't like that at all, and we both remember every single one of those classes with real fondness.

I couldn't actually sleep the night before the first class. I found it so exciting to think that I would be meeting so many women in the same situation as me and that I could probably talk freely about babies for two solid hours in the safe knowledge that I wouldn't be boring anyone!

The classes started at 8:00pm and finished at 10:00 pm. I would get our dinner prepared before we left so that it was all ready when we got home. It was always the same. Every week I would prepare a homemade pizza from scratch (all the dough and everything) with a big green salad. I knew that it was Jamie's favorite and it was sort of like a little thank you for making him endure the prenatal classes. Little did I know that he was secretly enjoying them – damn, I could have just used a premade pizza instead!

On the night of our first class, Jamie arrived back late from work (a recurring incident on Monday nights) so we rushed to try and get there by eight but not without getting lost first. The classes were held in a big house in Belsize Park and I had forgotten the number so we had to guess by the number of cars parked outside. We must have called on three houses, hand in hand, with my big pregnant belly, asking if we could come in; like Mary and Joseph looking for a room at the inn! The night was not starting off as I would have liked . . .

Finally, we found it and, as I suspected, we were the last couple to arrive. We were ushered into a large living room where we were met by 20 pairs of eyes and a deathly silence, broken only by the teacher expressing her annoyance that we had walked in with our shoes on (we were oblivious to the fact that there was a massive pile of shoes just outside the door). I instantly went a burning red – our hopes of just slipping nicely into the corner were dashed!

The first thing we were asked to do was find a partner and talk about ourselves for five minutes, so I turned to Jamie in the vain hope that no one would notice we had partnered up. But, of course, they had. This was another of my nightmares as it reminded me of my first day at school – a day that I would rather forget. However, I actually ended up talking to a very nice man named Barry. We chatted for five minutes or so and were then asked to tell the class about what we had just learned. NIGHTMARE. I hadn't even been listening – not because he wasn't interesting but because I was so nervous and wondering what task we would be set next. Oh God, this is not what I had imagined, and we had only been there 10 minutes. But as the class progressed we started to relax – this was obviously helped along by a task that I definitely approved of . . . your partner massaging you for five minutes. All that was missing was the whale music. Instead the silence was broken by little sniggers and giggles, mostly coming from the men (and one in particular!). It really did feel like school but I found this quite comforting and the two hours would fly by.

The one aspect of the class that I really enjoyed was when the group was split in half to discuss different subjects. The best ones were when the men were split up from the women and we would have girlie chats (mainly gossiping or moaning to each other about our husbands). It was always good fun, especially when we ended up talking about sex – it was like having a girls' night in. All that was missing was the giant bar of chocolate and the face masks! You might be wondering about the whole "sex during pregnancy" thing, and yes, this was one of the things we would end up discussing during our girlie chats!

My first comment would be, "What sex . . . ?" I am afraid that although some of you mad readers might be totally up for it, and want to know more, this will probably end up being a very short paragraph! Some pregnant women do end up feeling far more frisky when they are carrying a baby, due to all those raging hormones, but unfortunately for Jamie, I was one of those who just didn't want to know! It was as simple as that. A shame, though, as I think that Jamie fancied me more than ever when I was pregnant. I was just too frightened that we might accidentally knock the baby on its head – ridiculous I know, but a concern of mine nonetheless! Poor Jamie, as we ended up having our babies

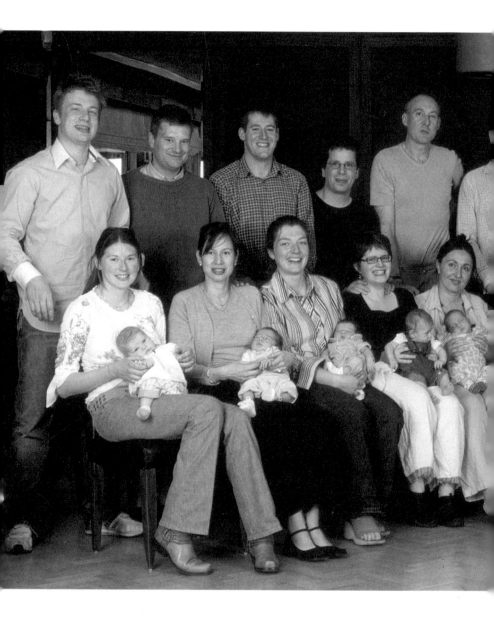

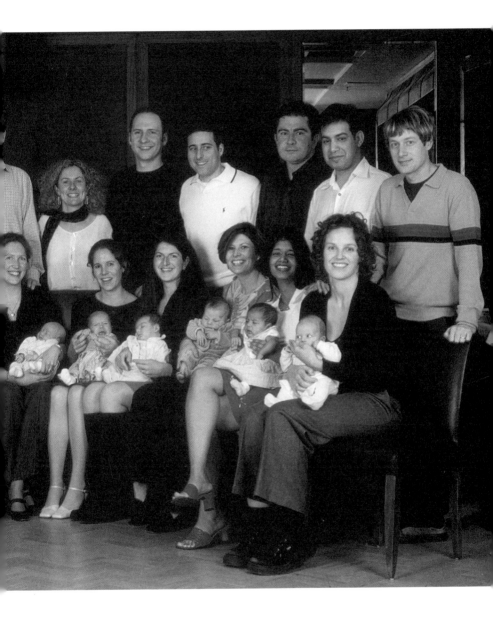

a year apart it meant that as soon as we were ready to get back in the saddle I was pregnant again. So unfortunately I can't give you any advice on what positions are best for sex when you're pregnant, but I say "go for it!" I later found out that it causes the baby absolutely no harm whatsoever, so when I get pregnant again in the future (fingers crossed), I will hopefully be able to put a smile back on Jamie's face for the whole nine months – let's wait and see!

The one thing in class that I was not keen on at all was the role playing. I would shrink like a potato chip bag in an oven when volunteers were required. Jamie would suddenly perk up and heckle everyone to choose me. One very brave girl (who has now become a close friend) was exceptionally good at it – especially when asked to simulate birth. I found her very convincing! I knew that I couldn't escape from it though, and one week found myself lying prostrate over an exercise ball pretending that I was 10 centimeters dilated and ready to push. What were they trying to do? Bring on an early labor? I was mortified and, naturally, redder than the Red Sea! Still, it amused Jamie.

Our lovely teacher, Ruth, was fantastic. She enjoyed a bit of role play and would often demonstrate the great uses of her fireplace by grabbing on to it and swaying through a particularly strong "contraction." Jamie and I would often joke that we bet her husband was a lucky man! The funny thing was, I did use her fireplace technique when I was in labor with Daisy and it was quite helpful. In fact, most of the things that we learned in the NCT classes followed us right the way through to labor. Jamie found himself shouting

Ruth's famous mantra with our first baby. It went something like this: "It's a life-giving pain; breathe through it; let it wash over you." At the time those words couldn't have meant less, but it made us laugh, and laughing through labor is a lot better than crying or pulling Jamie's hair out (more about that later!).

So, you can see, I really didn't know what to expect when we embarked on these classes. Confronted by my own self-consciousness and ten strangers with big bellies, the friendships and intimacy that arose were surprising, but so welcome. I think the main purpose was really to meet people in the same situation and basically bond over one of the most amazing things to ever happen to a couple. Some of them are still brilliant friends today. As a lot of my other friends have not had babies yet, it was really nice to be able to chat openly and honestly about the pregnancy. And then when you've had the baby, it's great to know that there are some people out there who understand what it's like because they are going through exactly the same thing. Having said that, the first impression that Jamie and I made (so my NCT mates tell me now) was rather bad. We were always the last to arrive and the first to leave. They thought we were stand-offish and unsociable – little did they know we were just bloody starving and desperate to go home and eat my homemade pizza!

LABOR BAGS AND BIRTH PLANS

Toward the end of your pregnancy you are advised (by books or your prenatal class) to have your birth plan written and your labor bag packed and ready to go so that if you go into labor suddenly, you are prepared. Unsurprisingly, I first came across the terms "labor bag" and "birth plan" when I was sifting through my many pregnancy and baby magazines. They really had dedicated quite a large section to the labor bag, so I thought it best that I pay great attention to what was required and, frankly, what the whole relevance of it was in the first place.

But first of all I had to put a birth plan together – here's what I wrote to take with me to the hospital (see opposite page).

So, with the birth plan prepared I now had to think about having a bag packed with a change of clothes, pajamas and a wash bag, then a separate bag with all the little things that your newborn baby will require, like onesies, diapers (a must!), cotton balls, maybe a teddy bear or two and, most importantly, his/her going home outfit!

The big question was: When should I pack my labor bag? My primary concern was that we were moving, and with all the upheaval and boxes, the last thing I wanted was to be rushing around mid-contraction looking for maternity pads! I didn't want to appear too eager, but then again I didn't want to tempt fate and leave it to the last minute. So, ever the organized mum-to-be, I started to pack my labor

Juliette Oliver's Birth Plan

Support
I would like my husband Jamie to be with me throughout the whole process of labour but I would also like my mum (Mrs Norton) to be there for extra support.

Positions for Labour
I would prefer to be in an upright position to work with gravity. I do have my own birthing ball which I have practised on to find a position that is good for me. It also helps with massage and backache, etc. Obviously this all depends upon how I'm feeling.

Pain Relief
I already have my TENS machine for the early stages of labour and hope to avoid any type of pain relief throughout labour. Obviously I'm not ruling out pain relief as I have no idea how I will feel, this being my first baby. I would, however, like to avoid any drugs that make you feel nauseous, sick or out of control and if I have an epidural I would like one which allows me to be mobile and walk around.

Caesarean Section
I would prefer to avoid a caesarean and try everything else before we resort to the c-section. But if the baby or myself are in any danger or distress we will take advice from my obstetrician. We will do whatever it takes to keep our baby and myself safe.

Monitoring the Baby
Being quite a nervous and anxious person, I would prefer to know that everything is well with the baby but I do not want to bring any unnecessary distress due to this intervention and I would prefer not to restrict my movement too long with the use of the belt, thus prolonging my labour. Again, we will do whatever it takes to keep our baby and myself safe and leave the ultimate decision to my obstetrician.

Delivery of the Placenta
I would like to be injected rather than have a natural delivery of the placenta. I know that this can be a quicker and safer process with few side effects.

bag two months before my due date! When it actually came to needing the bag, it was all dusty and cobwebby and had been bumped around during the move.

Did I fuss over this packing task or what? I went out and bought myself two new sports bags and deliberated for what felt like days over what to actually put in them. After reading countless articles and pamphlets giving advice, I decided to ignore them all and ended up packing half my wardrobe! For some reason I felt it completely necessary to pack every bit of medical paraphernalia under the sun. I also couldn't decide what to wear when I left the hospital or, for that matter, which pajamas and slippers I should take to wear in the hospital.

So, I thought that I would list all the things to show you what I packed for my first birth with Poppy. I have put an asterisk by all the items that I actually used. I'm a little embarrassed to show you my list now, as you'll think that I'm a little barmy, but I put all these decisions down to the hormones that were buzzing around my body at the time! Okay, here we go . . .

My Labour Bag

Clothes:

2 plain white t-shirts (not maternity ones, but a size 14 for that little extra room as I was unsure how much I would deflate post-baby but hoping that I would be back to my old size 10!) * I used one.

2 long-sleeved white t-shirts (same size) * I used one.

2 pairs of jeans (one maternity, the other a size 14 - again, living in hope)

1 pair of blue cords (not sure why I packed these but I just liked them)

1 pair of Topshop tracksuit bottoms (in lilac to match possible trainer in white with pink stripe) *

1 pair of white trainers with pink stripe *

1 pair of brown cowboy boots (Topshop, naturally!)

At this point I just want to stop and say, 'What was I thinking?' Trying to get cowboy boots on after you have just had a baby and second-degree stitches was absolutely impossible and, might I add, ridiculous!

2 pairs of socks * I used one.

6 pairs of white knickers * I used one.

12 pairs of maternity knickers in multicoloured polka dots (to detract from the fact that you are actually wearing aqua nappies!) *

Toiletries (thank God for Boots' loyalty cards)

1 spotty bag filled with brand new deodorant *
Facial wash *
Shower gel *
Moisturizer (day and night) *
Eye cream
Green spot cream for night time!
Toothbrush and paste *
Flannel *
Shampoo and conditioner *
Razor and shaving cream
Tweezers, mini scissors, eye lash curlers
Cotton wool
Maternity pads (VERY ESSENTIAL) x 4 bags *
Hairbrush and mini hairdryer
Straightening hair balm
Rescue remedy
Lavender bath oil
Neat tea tree oil
Arnica cream
Plasters (why on earth I felt I needed these I don't know... I was
   going to be in a hospital!)
Finally, moisturizer for my body and Cocoa Butter for stretch marks
   (fat lot of good)

Makeup:
Blemish cover up pot *
Under-eye concealer to hide BAGS (impossible at that stage)
Liquid blusher
Lip gloss in three colours
(I've never been a make-up person, so at least that was kept to
   a minimum!)

Extras

Birth plan (something you are advised to write but it didn't get
    referred to once during labour)
Hot and cold compresses
Various energy drinks and snacks
One of those plastic water bottles that professional cyclists use
A mini fan *
A face spray *
Massage oils and hand massager
Cards and Connect 4 (whatever!)
Vogue, Elle, Heat, Hello, OK, Now, New, Closer, Red, Cosmo and
    Glamour mags... My God, that list is just shocking.

And remember, I haven't even started on the baby's bag, although
(surprisingly,) I managed to keep it to a normal minimum (for me).
Here it is...

Baby Bag
(The bag was brand new from Nursery Window in Knightsbridge;
    seduced in the shop by the little pink rabbits on it!)
4 all-in-one suits with feet in white cotton and 2 in towelling * I used one.
4 white body suits with sleeves * I used one.
A going home outfit (which was, in fact, a white all-in-one) *
A gorgeous webbed baby blanket in white (which we wrapped Poppy up in
    when we left hospital. We kept it for Daisy too, and I think that I will
    offer it one day as a blanket for my grandchildren) *
A little woolly all-in-one for leaving the hospital (ours had little bear's ears — so
    sweet. Again, used for Daisy too.)
1 packet of newborn nappies *
1 bag of cotton wool and a baby bath sponge
A little duck rattle wrist band (she hated it!)

So there you have it. Quite a list. And I have to say it didn't stop there because there was my silver birthing/ exercise ball as well (which I consequently never even sat on throughout the whole labor). However, even though I didn't use it during labor it was still a damn good thing to have as I lolled about on it right through my pregnancy while reading a mag or watching TV. (Apparently, they are excellent for helping to get the baby down into your pelvis near your due date.) It was a hefty thing to carry to the car during labor, but with the ball packed away safely we really were giving Joan Collins a run for her money in the baggage stakes!

So much so that in our haste we forgot the most important thing to me: my little blanket which I have had since I was nine years old. It's called my "dankey" and was originally an Arsenal T-shirt which my dad had proudly presented to me when we planned to go to our first match together. He had a stroke soon after that so, sadly, that never happened but since then, wherever possible, I take that little bit of blanket everywhere with me. Twenty years later and it's now a scrap of material about the size of a golf ball. I didn't think that I could go through the birth without it because it feels like my strongest link to my wonderful dad who, I knew, would be by my side in spirit the whole way through. So it was inevitable that Jamie would have to drive home to get it once we were at the hospital!

It was hilarious to see just how much stuff I actually used from my labor bag and how much I didn't. It helped no end when I went into hospital again to have my second baby as I managed to cut my luggage in half . . . well, almost!

REACHING OUR DUE DATE

So, with the labor bag and birth plan all ready to go, there was just the little job of moving to our new house before I could go into labor! About a week or so before my due date I found myself standing in an empty house, the vacuum cleaner cord wrapped around my ankles and boxes piled high in the hallway. Our flat was now an empty little doll's house again and we were moving on. It felt only like yesterday that we were moving in as, ironically, my getting pregnant had coincided with us moving in nine months previously, and now we were leaving. I remember the first time we looked around the flat. It was snowing outside but so cozy inside – it felt like home immediately and I vividly recall the previous owner telling me to be careful about getting pregnant as she was four months pregnant and had a little toddler already without even intending to be a mum . . . fantastic, I thought. A flat with fertility powers – just what we needed! We loved that place and I can't even begin to tell you just how much effort and exertion we put into making that flat a home. It was the first place that we actually owned rather than rented (which we had done for the past seven years). So we felt that we could really go to town on the interior – as an example we had cowboy wallpaper in the bedroom and roses in the bathroom (heaven!). After being suppressed in our rented accommodations, we felt like we needed some artistic licence, although renting didn't ever stop Jamie. I remember in the "old" days when he was slightly less busy (I said only slightly), I would come home from a hard day of modeling and a night of waitressing and not only would he have cooked me a delish dinner but he'd also be down on his hands and knees laying Homebase linoleum tile on the matchbox-sized kitchen floor – the perfect husband-to-be I thought!

In our first studio flat, on Fitzjohn's Avenue in Hampstead, Jamie managed to fit one of those Victorian saucepan racks that attaches to the ceiling on a pulley system (Jamie is very good with his hands). In a kitchen that, I kid you not, was less than a meter square I thought we were living in a palace with the new linoleum down and the saucepans up above our heads! Our bed was on a loft above the sitting room and we literally had to crawl up a stepladder and could only crouch on the bed as it was so close to the ceiling. It was TINY, but we loved it. Many, many happy memories we have from that place.

Our second flat was on Humbolt Road in Hammersmith. It was a very dingy, dark basement flat, which Jamie and I shortly made into a little cozy haven with flowerpots going down the steps to brighten it up, and (once again) Homebase linoleum in the tiny kitchen! I loved it as I could ride my bike to my new waitressing job and back with Jamie in tandem – brilliant.

Our third flat was to become the set of the first ever *Naked Chef* series (the program that was to change our lives forever). I have to be honest, I hated it there, even though it was a hundred times bigger than anything I had ever dreamed that we would live in. But it was so cold and so different from what we were used to. And that spiral staircase! I'd try to slide down the banister too quickly to, say, get a nail file from the bedroom downstairs and would do myself a private injury!

The fourth flat, and possibly my favorite, was on Sumatra

Road in West Hampstead. It was a cute little one-bedroom flat with a garden that backed on to the railway. Naturally, it wasn't long before we had laid the Homebase linoleum and erected the saucepan rack and I loved it there. It felt like a real home – aside from the rats in the garden and the drunk man in the basement flat downstairs! From there we moved to the hotel at Monte's, then on to Gardnor Road in Hampstead which is where I was standing that morning, nine months pregnant and feeling highly emotional!

The Olivers being the Olivers, we thought that we could move into our new house unaided, apart from a little help from our friends and a white van. It didn't seem to register with my husband that I was about to give birth and that moving to a new house and having a baby are up there as two of the most stressful things you can do in life! But maybe the fact that I was pregnant and probably at the pinnacle of my "Monica" stage and raring to go helped that cause somewhat! So, with nearly all our boxes loaded on to the van, we were ready to move up the road.

Up to now I've talked about all the things that can happen to the body of a pregnant woman, but I'm still not sure what happens psychologically. Near the end of my pregnancy, I turned almost animalistic when it came to cleaning and organizing things. We had exactly one week to make this new house a home. According to my dates, Poppy was due on March 13 and, being naive and inexperienced I thought that she would be here on that date, come hell or high water! So I took it upon myself to bring her home to a pristine, clean, beautiful palace.

Maybe it was just me, but as I scrubbed and swept, bleached and unpacked, everyone else around me was . . . involved in doing a photo shoot. What? Was Jamie mad? He had strategically planned a shoot in our house for a food magazine where he was to cook sausages in our new Aga oven. Arrrrrrgh! I was furious, and even more furious than I would have been if I hadn't been pregnant. As my sister and I, with my best friend Jim lounging on the floor, were grappling with the baby's cradle in the nursery, surrounded by screws and instructions, something boiled up inside me and I just exploded with anger. I stormed down the stairs and into the living room and raged as I watched Jamie and about seven media magazine types *oooing* and *ahhing* like spectators at a fireworks display. They were all munching on sausages, and I let rip as only a hormonal nine-months-pregnant woman could! I think I shouted something like "where are my bloody sausages, you selfish *******?" Now this is totally, totally out of character for me and I cringe at the mere thought that I actually had the guts to say it, but when you think about it I probably could have said a lot worse. It worked, you know. I have never seen so many people (and especially Jamie) swallow down their food and jump up to assist me in all my life. It was fabulous!

Believe it or not, by 7:00 that night, our house was finished. Every box, except for two, had been unpacked, and the kettle was on. Jamie was safely ensconced at work (much to his relief) and I took some time out for the first time that day. I lay in the nursery listening to our baby's music mobile, relishing every moment of our new life and our new beginning as a soon-to-be family of three. I was excited beyond belief! And as I checked out each room, I happily came to the conclusion that I could proudly enter it into the next homes and gardens mag – it was that tidy! With that settled, I curled up in our new sitting room and watched *Sex and the City* and secretly thanked Pops for not coming early.

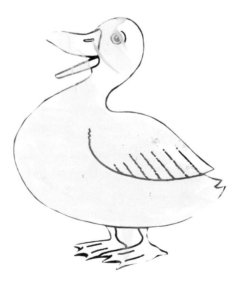

CHAPTER FIVE

Labor, Delivery and Breastfeeding

NO PAINKILLERS FOR ME...

The labor bit was always the first chapter that I would turn to in all the books I had on pregnancy. I thought that it was one of the most exciting and intriguing parts of this whole baby process. Now, of course, neither of these words immediately springs to mind when I think back!

I have to admit, I wasn't the least bit scared about actually giving birth because I had really only heard very positive things about it. I had all but exhausted my mum with my countless requests to give me every detail of when she gave birth to me and my two sisters – not that she minded, as I think she loved telling us all about it. Mum gave birth to all three of us naturally and with absolutely no pain relief at all. With my eldest sister, Nathalie, she was in labor for a total of about nine hours and managed to read a copy of *Vogue* magazine before she popped her out (that might explain Nat's penchant for the mag!). With Lisa, the second eldest, Mum had a relaxing bath and, before she knew it, Lee was making her way into the world. When it came to me, she didn't even make it into the hospital – I decided to arrive within the comfort of our house which, naturally, had my dad running around like a headless chicken trying to keep calm. The way my mum describes it, it sounded like he was one of those typical dads you see in the movies who bolts out the door and jumps into the car to drive to the hospital when the first contraction arrives, leaving their delirious partner stranded at the front door! Apparently, in the midwife's dash to get to the house in time she managed to drive over my dad's pristine lawn and through the flowers, which had him literally pulling his hair out. I don't know why he bothered – in my experience (all will be revealed . . .), I am sure Mum could have done that for him!

Upon the midwife's arrival, she sternly asked my dad to put the kettle on as she dashed upstairs. Dad touchingly asked if she required milk and sugar with her tea and at that she retorted, "Not for me, you idiot – some hot water for your wife as she is about to give birth!" And then I arrived!

I loved hearing Mum tell these stories. To me it all sounded like fun – and quite easy. I was looking forward to reading the latest issue of *Elle* magazine and then popping the baby out. Yes, this was going to be a great challenge but, of course, as easy births obviously run in our family I was going to do it without pain relief, too. Cue the birth day!

However, the first time I started to have doubts about this labor lark was when I heard Jamie's sister, Anna, having contractions for her second baby. We were both pregnant at the same time and, luckily for me, she was due two months before me, so I relied on her to give me all the ins and outs (literally) of her birth. Anna had also had a lovely first labor with absolutely no pain relief, so I was expecting the same for her this time. Jamie and I had just polished off our usual Saturday afternoon fish and chips at our local west London hot spot when we received the phone call that we had been waiting for – Anna was in labor. Fantastic (or so I thought)! The screams I heard in the background were really scary, and I wondered what she was doing. Why was she shouting? It couldn't be that bad, surely? Her labor was great in the end, but not without a lot of screaming at her husband, Paul, to put his foot down in the car or she would have had her second son, James, on the Addenbrooke's Hospital roundabout in Cambridge!

(It's just dawned on me that I've written a couple of pages on labor and delivery without even touching on my own. That's because – I can't emphasize this enough! – I'd become obsessed with hearing about everyone else's.)

One day I happened across the Discovery Health Channel on television – nonstop programming about health issues, mainly focusing on real-life pregnancy and birth stories, showing women in labor and actually giving birth! That was it! I had this channel on all the time – hourly, daily, nightly. I found it all so fascinating and it really helped to open my eyes to the amount of different labor experiences that women have. (And they were not all like my mum's, I can tell you!) I learned so much from watching these programs – they were real eye-openers . . .

I could sense the annoyance in Jamie when at 6:20 am the opening credits for the program would start – even the title music got on his nerves. His pillow would instantly go over his head and then I would be ushered downstairs to watch television in the sitting room.

HOW CLEAN WAS OUR HOUSE?

Leading up to my due date, I was sure that our baby would be early, but with each day that passed after my due date I got more and more agitated. Why wasn't the baby coming? Was I going to be pregnant forever? My cleaning obsession had gone into overdrive because each day I thought that it would be the day I was going to bring a baby home and I wanted the house to be the most pristine-sterile-spotless-shining-fresh-laundry-smelling abode! Even I can admit that I was turning into a nightmare. I constantly wore a pair of rubber gloves – they were like my second skin. They were definitely my favorite accoutrements – not far behind were the Dettox disposable wipes, the Parazone flushable toilet cleaning wipes and the Pledge polish. And don't forget the vacuum cleaner . . . lugging that around was a sight to see when I was nine months pregnant, but oh so necessary!

I became irritated by absolutely any mess whatsoever. Poor Jamie couldn't even move in the house for fear of being mopped into oblivion. Resistance was futile. He even stopped shoving his socks behind the sofa – results!

This happened with both my pregnancies. When I was 10 days overdue with my second daughter, Daisy, my cleaning habits went through the roof. I had become so irritated with our sofa in the sitting room because it, rather appropriately, gave birth to mini feathers every day, that one of the jobs I just HAD take care of (it's weird what goes through your head when you're pregnant!) was to have the sofa recushioned.

Anyway back to giving birth to our first baby . . .

"BY THURSDAY, WE'LL BE PARENTS...!"

I was now two days past my due date and Jamie and I were going for a routine check-up with our obstetrician at the hospital. I don't know why but I thought that he would have all the answers to my incessant questions like:

"What day exactly do you think the baby will arrive?"

"How much will he/she weigh?"

"In fact, what sex is it? Can you tell by the way I am carrying?"

Of course he didn't know the answers to any of these things (just yet anyway). But he was sure that we should only wait until we were seven or eight days past our due date before we talked about being induced. I remember listening to what he was saying and trying to take it all in, when suddenly it hit me – he had said that if the baby hadn't arrived at a certain time I would be induced and that I should have the baby definitely by next Thursday. Oh my God – we'd been given a date! Finally it became real. I now knew that by Thursday, at the very latest, Jamie and I would be parents. It was both very exciting and very scary.

I was determined to try and get this baby out without having to wait to be induced. I wanted him or her sooner than that – I had waited nine long months for this after all! So Jamie and I set to work at getting our little one out. I tried all the usual techniques that frustrated overdue women try.

There was the extremely hot curry . . . but no delivery (only the delivery of searing heartburn which I could well have done without!).

Then I tried eating pineapple. I had seen it on one of the many TV shows that I had watched – it was meant to help with bringing on the birth (but God knows how . . . it's only a fruit!).

Jamie seemed to visibly perk up at one of the midwife's suggestions of – wait for it – SEX! Was she mad? That really was the last thing I wanted to be trying at this stage. Maybe the baby could stay in for a little while longer after all!

It was getting to the point where friends would be calling up anxious for some news and, down in the village, people would stop us and the usual comment would be, "Haven't you had it yet?" Arrrrrgh – did it look like I had had it?

Well, finally the day arrived. I mean, I didn't know it but I knew something strange was in the air. Jamie headed off to Borough Market as he usually does on a Saturday morning. I asked him not to be too long, as you never know. (I had said this every day for the last month, so I had a feeling that his reassurance that he wouldn't be long held no weight!) Naturally, I wasn't the only one who was well overdue. Jamie must have gotten lost amongst the dried fruit and sensational array of fresh herbs because he didn't make it back home until well in the afternoon. I was furious when he finally arrived – all smiles and laden down with his precious produce. What was he thinking? I could have given birth by now. I mean, the fact that I hadn't meant nothing to me – in my mind I was in the hospital on my own, pushing for dear life.

When Jamie then suggested that we go down to the local pet shop to get some fish for our pond (as a little outing to get me out of the house), I think I totally flipped out. Was he completely bonkers? I don't know whether it was because I was hungry, tired and fed up or whether my hormones were kicking in and I was starting labor. I thought it was the latter as behavior like that is totally out of character for me (and I know that Jamie will agree). As I sobbed on the nursery floor, willing the baby to just come, she must have heard my call as only hours after my tantrum, at about 6:30 that evening, I went to the bathroom and there was the first positive sign that I could be in labor . . . I had had a "show"! If you're not sure what a show is, then all I shall say here is that it is also called a "mucus plug" – you can either leave it up to your imagination or have a look at the glossary on page 285 to read a bit more about it! I dashed downstairs to Jamie and he said that I was as white as a sheet. Just as I told him what had happened he started to tuck into his lamb dinner! He looked a little confused – I mean, why would a man understand the great importance of a show?

From that point on, I was a bundle of excitement and nerves. I called the maternity ward countless times to track my progress with them – I'm sure they were all overjoyed to hear that Mrs. Oliver Was Now in Labor. Classically, I ignored everything I had read and learned at the NCT classes. I thought that our baby would arrive by morning and was desperate to go to the hospital to get myself organized and settled.

I decided to pass on my dinner that night (a big mistake, as this would have been my last meal for 48 hours) but I was paranoid that I would have a heavy stomach which would in turn make me feel sick. Instead I had a warm bath and decided to preen myself for labor. I washed my hair, shaved, plucked, waxed and creamed – I really was ready to receive my little baby. Oh, and the midwives and doctors were ready to receive her too, thanks to my immaculate bikini line!

As I got into bed, I could feel the onset of contractions and by three in the morning I had Jamie up timing them. They were still 10 minutes apart so we decided to watch a film – we both ended up in stitches watching *Dude, Where's My Car?* At 5:00 am there was still no baby! Of course, by morning we were both drained and exhausted as we hadn't had any sleep. Stupid really because although I'd had steady contractions throughout the night, they were hardly painful; just like mini-period pains. We both regretted staying up when sleeping is what we should have been doing in order to make it through the day, as we had NO idea what was in store for us!

By midday, and my third bath in as many hours, the contractions started to gather pace. I called my mum who came straight over. She hadn't seen our new house before, so Jamie was showing her around while I yelled out my contraction timings from the sitting room. They were still only every 10 minutes – what was going on? It felt like I should be having the baby NOW! As the day progressed I noticed that I had started to bleed a lot more than I thought was usual. Apart from the show, I had seemed to bleed steadily throughout the day so I became a bit concerned that something was wrong. Was this normal? I called the delivery ward and after they reassured me that this was a normal process of labor I decided to try, for the first time since this all began, to relax!

Jamie was looking forward to looking after my mum by cooking a delicious roast chicken. As he set about preparing the feast, I tried to ignore my growing contractions. After some time I couldn't stand it any longer – I wanted to get to a hospital and FAST! So, with the giant bouncy ball, my countless labor bags, a reticent Jamie (who was still concerned about the progress of his roast chicken in the oven) and a groaning me in tow, we all set off for the hospital in Hammersmith.

Once we'd arrived, I was convinced that I was close to giving birth but, after a swift examination, I found that I was still only 1 centimeter dilated . . . WHAT? It couldn't be true – according to my pain threshold I should be about to start pushing right now! I wondered how many women go into the hospital with this same feeling and find out they are way off giving birth, just like me.

As we all sat in the hospital room, I noticed that Jamie had a concerned look on his face. I tried to reassure him that although it looked like I was in hell, really I was okay and he was not to worry. As he held my hand with a furrowed brow he said, "Babe, I am not worried about you – you are doing brilliantly. It's just that my chicken is in the Aga and it looks like we are in for a long night. Should I go home and refuel so I can support you later on when you need it?" What can I say? It was probably a good time to have suggested something so ridiculous because in my state I would have let him jump out of a plane!

So, it was just Mum and me and the company of the TV to pass the time. By ten o'clock that night, I hadn't dilated any further. Jamie returned to the hospital looking refreshed and replenished – lucky bastard. I felt anything but! The pain of each contraction was hitting me hard and I found myself hanging on to the metal bedstead for support, gritting my teeth during each wave of pain (this wasn't good; I didn't know that it would feel like this). At four in the morning, after yet another internal to check my dilation and impromptu water break (exactly how you imagine the gushing of water flooding out . . . it felt like Niagara Falls down there), I finally relented and begged the midwife for some sort of pain relief. Well, this certainly wasn't in the birth plan . . .

The first thing I was offered was "gas and air" through a mask which I promptly threw across the room after just two inhalations. I thought it was hideous and it made me feel worse than before. Plus, the room was now spinning! With Jamie's wrist now resembling the aftermath of a Chinese burn competition, we both decided that an epidural was the only answer. I was just too tired to go without but at the same time I was so disappointed in myself. In my haze of pain I remember asking the midwife if any of the other ladies on the ward were having an epidural. I obviously didn't want to be the odd one out (the things you think about in some situations!). I had asked for a mobile epidural as this would dull the pain completely but also allow me to walk about if I wanted to.

Naturally, as soon as the anesthetist had administered my epidural I told him I was in love with him and asked if I could marry him! I wonder how many marriage proposals and declarations of love this man has received since starting the job – I suspect quite a few! My adoration for him was heightened by the fact that he really was my big support. For some reason, while the injection was being prepared, my husband seemed to have disappeared. It was only after a couple of minutes that I noticed a pair of sneaker-clad feet standing neatly behind the curtain. What on earth was Jamie doing behind there? His fear of needles had resurfaced, and the size of this one made him feel a little queasy – this was coming from a man who has deboned whole pigs for a living. Classic!

Once the epidural took effect, I felt fabulous. It was amazing to think that only minutes ago I had been gripped with pain and now my body was dealing with these contractions on its own and I couldn't even feel them! I finally relaxed and allowed myself to fall asleep. When I woke at 7:00 the next morning I wondered where I was. It was like waking up on Christmas morning and finding that Father Christmas hadn't delivered your Christmas presents!

I was offered breakfast, but I still couldn't face any food so I passed it on to Jamie who, by now, was looking completely exhausted, having slept rather uncomfortably in the chair next to me. I managed a couple of sips of tea and even a bite of one of those hideous energy bars that I had insisted on packing in my labor bag. We were both feeling a bit fed up now. Apparently during the night my contractions had slowed down considerably as a result of the epidural (sometimes this can happen if you have an epidural). I felt like our baby was never going to arrive. As time ticked slowly on, I started to worry that as I was dilating so slowly I could end up having a caesarean. I was worried that the midwives and doctors would only give me a little more time but I really believed that I could do this on my own, and I wanted to do it on my own. As Jamie and I cuddled up on the bed watching Monday morning TV, the midwives and doctors kept coming in to monitor me and the baby. I'd become very used to being prodded and pulled in all directions by this point.

By about midday, I could tell that Jamie was starting to get fidgety – we really had not expected it to take so long, no matter how many times we were told by various friends and NCT teachers! I think it was down to lack of food – typical! (Thank God I allowed him to have that roast chicken. I dread to think what state he would have been in by this point.) After much begging, I allowed Jamie out of my sight to call for a pizza delivery, but I'd started to feel incredibly sick – this was the last thing I needed now, especially as Jamie had insisted on ordering my favorite margarita pizza but with anchovies (which I told him that I would NEVER eat in a month of Sundays right now).

Again Jamie had to resume his hiding place behind the curtain while he ate the pizza and salad with dough balls. I couldn't even stand the smell at this point. Admirably allowing him to finish his long-awaited lunch, I finally relented and was sick not just once, but three times; each time with Jamie holding one of those hospital bedpan trays out for me as a bowl, trying to make me laugh at the same time. By this time I had begun to feel thoroughly sorry for myself. Where was my bundle of joy and my *Vogue* magazine?

We were watching *Richard and Judy* when the midwife told us the news that we had been waiting for . . . I was almost 10 centimetres dilated and would be ready to push within the hour. Yeaaahhhhhh! What a relief to hear that news. When the time came to push it was obviously hard because I had no feeling from the epidural, and no inclination to push, so taking the midwife's lead and under her instruction I started to push for dear life. It really was the strangest sensation as I couldn't feel a thing; even my legs were numb.

The midwife and my obstetrician were able to tell when I was having a contraction through the monitor that I was linked up to and with each wave of a contraction they chorused me to PUSHHHHH. It was so weird. But that really wasn't a problem. The problem was just to the left of me in the form of my husband, as he hoisted my leg up in the air and insisted that I would be in a better position if I stood up and leaned over the bed. Now, this was all very well and good but I had had an epidural and I couldn't feel anything from the waist down, so how the hell was I supposed to stand up? With this idea promptly put to bed, Jamie quickly came up with another one. "How about if I put Jools' leg over my shoulder and . . ."

"HOW ABOUT YOU MOP MY BROW AND FAN ME DOWN?!"

But for Jamie, who obviously felt like he was orchestrating service on a busy night at the restaurant, that wasn't enough. He preferred to be down the dodgy end assisting the doctor, so as I looked down I now had two pairs of expectant eyes willing me to PUSH! On further examination our obstetrician realized that the baby was coming out sideways, which can make for a more painful and difficult birth. There was suddenly talk of using a vacuum to aid the delivery which I was slightly worried about. This is a piece of medical equipment like a big pair of suction-operated tongs and

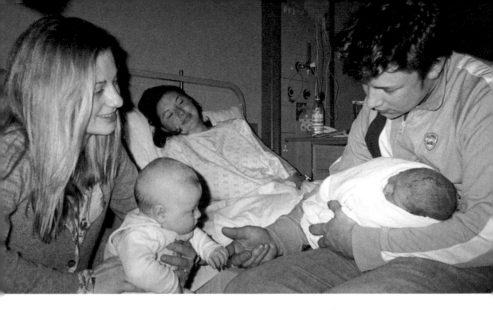

it's used to help pull the baby out if there is a chance that it might get stuck in the birth canal. I wasn't all that into it but, again, if it meant that the baby would be safe I didn't mind.

After what felt like hours, but it was in fact only one, our beautiful baby daughter, Poppy, was born. It was incredible – she was quickly passed to me wrapped in a blanket. I lay her on top of me so we both had our skin touching and she opened her eyes and stared at us without uttering a single cry. It was magical. I really can't remember anything else, just the way that Poppy smelled. The rest is a wonderful haze of happiness. Poppy Honey Rosie Oliver had finally arrived.

X

BREASTFEEDING

With the labor out of the way and Poppy safe and sound, the very first thing I had to contend with was breastfeeding. Now this is quite a long section, as there's quite a lot to say, so I'm going to tackle it all in one go and then take you back into the story, with us leaving hospital and our first few days at home at the start of the next chapter. I hope that's okay!

I had always wanted to breastfeed our babies, and I think that this was due to the fact that I didn't know any different. My sisters and I were all breastfed and so were Jamie and his sister, Anna. And now my eldest sister Nat was breastfeeding too. So it seemed natural for me to do the same. I thought that it looked incredibly easy and a wonderful thing to do, so as I got nearer and nearer to my due date with Poppy it was definitely one of the things I was most looking forward to.

We were lucky at our prenatal group as we were offered an extra class exclusively about breastfeeding. At first I thought that it would be pointless to learn about breastfeeding when you didn't actually have your baby to practice with, but nonetheless I signed up for it. I thought it best to at least try; after all I still didn't have a clue how to do up a sleeper, let alone feed my baby! So off I went. The class was packed, with all the NCT girls gathered round in the usual semicircle. It was weird not having any of the men there – it was more relaxed and comfortable (after all, if I was going to be getting my boobs out I would rather it be with just the girls, thank you very much!). It was all very

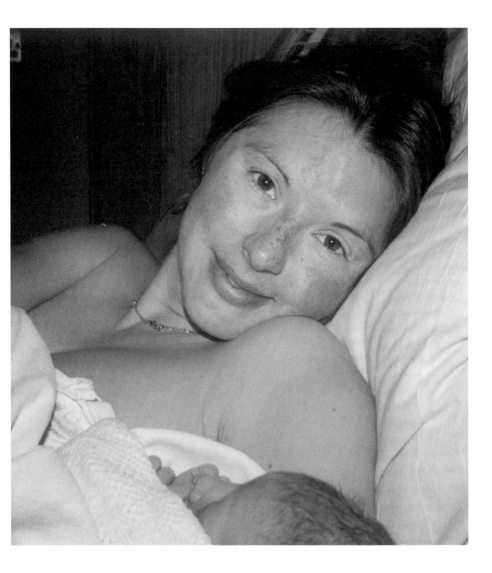

helpful; even using little plastic dolls as our future babies I learned a lot.

I was very shocked to learn that breastfeeding actually involves some quite skilled maneuvering. I just thought it was a matter of putting your baby to your nipple and letting her do the rest! Of course it could never be that simple. There is a specific technique you have to learn in order to get your baby to "latch on" successfully. It's all about angles really and letting your baby take charge! At the prenatal class we were given a diagram to show us how to hold the baby to the nipple and so, armed with my plastic baby and the diagram, I set about practicing my nearly acquired skill.

Okay, enough practicing. It was now time for the real thing. As soon as Poppy was born, she was handed to me. I laid her on my chest and within minutes she was foraging for my breast. I was shocked at her eagerness, as I hadn't anticipated that. With a bit of fumbling she was on . . . no, wait a minute, she was off again. Hang on. She was a lot harder to manipulate than my plastic baby who had seemed to latch on perfectly first time and stay there for hours! With Poppy falling on and off my boob, I decided to give in and relax. After all, I had just given birth and was too tired at this point to worry about breastfeeding. And obviously Pops wasn't too concerned because she fell asleep as well.

Undeterred by my first attempt and now back in the comfort of our little room in the ward, it was just me and Poppy, this time with no overzealous audience peeking in or (God forbid) tweaking my nipples to try and help the process along! For the first time since she had been born, I was now in charge and alone. I had been given a special typed-up sheet by the midwife, which had a chart to help me with my breastfeeding times. Apparently, I was to feed Poppy on one breast first and then write down which one I had chosen. Then on the next feed I was supposed to put her on the other breast. That sounded simple enough. It didn't say how long I was supposed to keep her on the boob but, hey, maybe I should be thinking for myself on this one. It was beginning to feel like school!

The second time I breastfed Poppy was much better. She seemed to latch on fairly quickly and, from what I could tell, she was content with her first proper meal! It only lasted about five minutes though (naturally I was timing the feeds to add to the worksheet – after all I wanted to receive top marks from the chief midwife on the ward. I wanted to be their best student!).

Okay. Feed number three. "Shit! Where's my pen and work sheet?" as Poppy's screams reverberated through the ward during the middle of the night. I was trying to weigh my boobs with my hand, wondering which one was heaviest, and attempting to tally that up with my worksheet. "Bugger," I thought. So I decided to go with the left boob and on Poppy went again with no trouble. I had a pillow propped underneath my arm and Pops was laying on it clamped to my breast. I marveled at the sudden quietness that ensued (as I am sure every other new mum does too)! And with only a flickering TV in the background for company, I fell asleep in a state of bliss.

What was all this fuss about cracked nipples and sore boobs that we were warned about at NCT? Mine felt fabulous! And, may I say, Jamie thought they looked pretty good too! Now, remember, I am only talking day two here. By the time we had taken Poppy home for the first time and settled into a kind of breastfeeding routine, suddenly the pain everyone had talked about set in. Firstly, I noticed that every time Poppy fed from me I had the most searing pain like a crunching sensation in my stomach. It felt as if I had a very tight clamp strapped to my lower tummy, pulling tighter every time she sucked. At first I thought that maybe I had eaten something dodgy at the hospital, but once she had stopped feeding the pain ebbed away almost as fast as it had arrived. After a chat with my midwife she explained that breastfeeding helps the uterus to contract and that was what I was feeling. Perfect, I thought. At least that sorted out the first problem and as time went on the nagging feeling subsided. After about two weeks it had gone completely and I didn't feel it again.

My next hurdle was incredibly painful, cracked nipples. They really were a sight. Every time Pops clamped her little gums and mouth on to the nipple, I gave a yelp of pain if I was alone in the room and sometimes sat there crying with pain. I really had to grit my teeth as Poppy went at it. I often found myself stamping my feet and grunting like a pig to deal with it. In fact, every time she fed from me I got myself into a grunting and stamping routine (much to the distress and disgruntlement of Jamie or whoever else was in the room at the time)! But the torture only lasted about a minute and as soon as she was settled there we both relaxed.

A good tip which my sister-in-law Anna-Marie gave me was not to slather my nipples in specialized nipple cream but to allow them to dry and crack as this way they would become hardened to it and within weeks they would heal. I did as she advised and it worked, although it's thoroughly tempting to coat yourself in cream, especially if it has been in the fridge for a while as it can be a really instant soother. Try both ways and see which works for you. I do remember, especially in those early days, sitting cross-legged on the floor in our sitting room with my tracksuit bottoms on and one of Jamie's shirts completely opened to the waist with no bra on. I sat eating my dinner with Poppy clamped to one boob and I held a bag of petit pois on the other exposed breast. What a sight, but at the time it was the norm and my mum and Jamie certainly weren't going to complain (I don't think they would have dared!).

I actually found feeding Poppy the regular way (in the cradle position) quite hard to master at first so my midwife showed me a different, more effective way for me by using one of those specialized boomerang-shaped cushions which I could place around my waist and then put Poppy into position under my arm (it's called the rugby ball position because it looks like you're carrying a rugby ball!). This seemed to work brilliantly and I soon became reliant on my super-sized boomerang cushion. I even called up my health visitor to ask if it would ever be possible for me to feed Poppy without using it as I imagined going for coffee with my NCT pals and whipping out my cushion!

For the first few days after giving birth the only milk supply that you have is called "colostrum." It's a yellowish color, and has the texture of skimmed milk as it's very watery. This milk is filled with all the essential nutrients that newborns need. I didn't actually get my proper milk coming in until about four days after Poppy was born. I had almost forgotten that it would be arriving and so was quite shocked to wake up one night to find massive wet patches circling my boobs and a completely wet sheet. I couldn't figure out what had happened and thought that in my catatonic state I had poured water on myself from my glass on the side table. As I sat up, I felt this strange sensation in my breasts. They were incredibly painful and heavy like you wouldn't believe. They were massive and as hard as rocks; they even felt bumpy to touch . . . So this is what they meant when they talked about your milk coming in!

My instinct told me that I had to empty these and fast. I couldn't bear to wake Poppy up to feed her so I decided that I would have to extract it myself. Luckily I had read up on this chapter when I was pregnant – hand expressing, I think it was called. It was simple enough (I know that I could have just tried to use my breast pump, as this situation was exactly what they were designed for, but at three in the morning I was in NO mood to deal with the instructions). What I should have done is bought my breast pump well in advance and read the instructions so I knew what to do. Anyway, I went off to the bathroom and hand expressed some of my new milk. This was so fascinating! I was basically kneading my boobs from the outside in and the milk was coming out so fast. The relief it brought me was almost instant. At some points I didn't even have to push it out as it flowed out on its own. This only happened every so often; especially if Poppy had had a day where she ate little. My milk supply would be overflowing, as she wasn't a great guzzler.

My breast pump often came in handy as I would just express the excess milk and either freeze it or throw it away. I would do this more frequently when weaning Poppy as she got older. I'll talk about this in more detail later, but as soon as Poppy had sampled real food, her intake of my milk lessened and it was inevitable that I was going to have this huge excess of wasted milk. At times it was just too painful to ignore. It got confusing, though, because I was also told that if I expressed too much, my milk supply would increase. I felt like I was in a little bit of a no-win situation, but the odd breast pump here and there was okay as long as it was to get rid of excess milk (it's beginning to sound like an addiction . . . you wait and see for yourself because quite frankly it is!).

It always made us laugh when I put Poppy on the breast first thing in the morning when my supply was at its greatest. There is a process called the "let-down reflex" where the milk rushes from your milk glands to your nipple, and if Poppy happened to fall off my boob the milk would spray out like a fine shower all over her face. If I hadn't been paying attention for a couple of minutes, I'd look down and see her little face covered in milk!

Now, the only way to stop all these wet mattresses, sheets, pajamas and clothes is to wear breast pads. I hated them, so I rejoiced when it was no longer necessary to have them and gleefully chucked the whole supply in the trash. Basically they are like sanitary napkins for boobs – what more can I say? But they were exceedingly helpful, especially in the early stages of breastfeeding when leakage was just par for the course. It is advised that you wear them at night, but for me they were just too irritating. I would often find rogue pads in the strangest of places – under the bed, behind the sofa and in Poppy's toy box of all places. They seemed to have minds of their own! It was never amusing to have a nice day out and find that, once you got home and looked in the mirror, your boob pads had been showing quite prominently all day through your T-shirt. Two circular eyes peering out of your chest – now, that's attractive!

I was initially surprised at how little Poppy drank during the day. She always seemed to be asleep but, of course, it was a completely different story during the night. For the very first few nights of Poppy's life, being woken up by her every few hours was a pleasure. We used to lie awake watching her little body – arms splayed out above her head – and will her to wake up so we could cuddle her and then, as soon as she stirred, we would whip her out of her cradle. Jamie and I would both be vying for her attention and, of course, I would always win as I was the meals on wheels! Until week two . . . yes, it only took about 14 days for us both (well, me especially) to realize that sleep deprivation was killing us!

Instead of lying awake willing Poppy to wake up, I would lie rigid in my bed praying for her to stay asleep. As soon as I heard the familiar little noises coming from the cradle, I knew she was stirring. My heart would beat faster as I hoped it was just a mere murmur and not the full-on three-course

meal beckoning! But, of course, within minutes she would be screaming her head off and I would have her out of her cradle quicker than lightning in case she woke Jamie up.
I found these feeds incredibly hard. In fact, if I'm being honest, the words I would use to describe them are "pure punishment." I couldn't believe that in two weeks I had gone from feeling pleasure to punishment. How could this be? I was doing three feeds a night (approximately midnight, 3:00 am and 6:00 am) and found the midnight one the hardest to deal with. Having gone to bed at nine, I would instantly fall into a deep, luxurious sleep only to be woken abruptly and put straight into action. My body was in shock!

Propped up against my pillows with Poppy attached to my boob, happily sucking away, I would feel my eyes getting heavier and heavier and would end up dozing off. It felt like it was only for a couple of seconds but when I looked at the clock I would realize that in fact an hour had passed and Poppy had fallen asleep too. I would carefully place her back in her cradle, but no matter how careful I was as soon as she was on her mattress her eyes would open and the look she gave me spoke volumes. I could have handled the look but it was the cry that followed which I couldn't fight! So, there we were again – me propped up staring into space like a zombie and Poppy back where she loved in the warmth of my breast. And as I looked over to my left there was Jamie sleeping like … a baby! I really don't know which was more frustrating – the peaceful and relaxed sleeping Jamie or the incessant waking and feeding of Poppy. I had started to resent Jamie and thought, how dare he be enjoying his sleep when I couldn't. Of course this was not a rational thought. You have to trust me; when you haven't slept properly for weeks you start to go a little insane. God forbid if he started to snore mid-feed; I think I might have killed him. When I look back now, I want to laugh just thinking about the dagger eyes I would give him if he gently tried to stroke my back in sympathy whilst he made those unmistakable sleeping coos . . . it's not fair!

As cringeworthy as it is to reveal this, on really bad nights when I struggled to stay awake and keep my patience as little Poppy fed for hours on end, I used to make a very big fuss about getting her up and feeding her. I don't always think it was completely necessary to turn all the lights on in the bedroom or have the TV on for company in the background, but sometimes you just feel like the only person in the world who is awake in what seems like a very lonely place!

I remember on one of these particular nights, when I was up feeding my second daughter, Daisy, I was watching *Dallas* on UK Gold (I say watching – I was actually rocking Daisy back and forth around the room trying to soothe her while catching glimpses of Sue Ellen and JR snogging after another drunken fight!) when my mobile phone beeped with a text message. It was from my friend Lindsey who had also just had her little baby, Joel. She was up breastfeeding him at that ungodly hour and it was brilliant to know that there was someone else out there in exactly the same situation – it certainly helped to keep me awake!

LET'S GET INTO A ROUTINE

After a few weeks I managed to get myself into a regular daytime routine with Poppy and her feeding times, as I had decided not to feed on demand. I was quite surprised at first, when Poppy was newborn, that not every cry was for food, as I assumed that that's the only thing she would want. I hadn't a clue what else she would need. However, you soon learn that it could be a dirty diaper or gas which meant that Poppy needed burping.

Once I had mastered all these other checks, if she was still crying I would then put her on the breast. On one particularly fraught morning my mum showed me that perhaps a little cuddle and a walk around the room would be just as satisfactory as putting her on the breast, and at once she relaxed and stopped crying. Seeing this allowed me to learn to establish a good routine of my own that worked for me. It involved feeding her approximately every four hours, with the first feed at around 7:00 am, then 11:00 am, 3:00 pm and finally 7:00 pm. Of course, at first none of these times were guaranteed, especially if we had had a bad night. I just tried to stick to some sort of routine that felt natural to both Poppy and me. I know all babies are different, but this is what worked for me. After only a few months she had it figured out and I started to feel a bit more ordered in my head.

Not feeding her on demand also allowed me to realize that in between the feeds, the cries and agitation would be due to something else. It was so illuminating when I worked out that Poppy had different cries for communicating different things to me. I know that it sounds a bit like mumbo jumbo

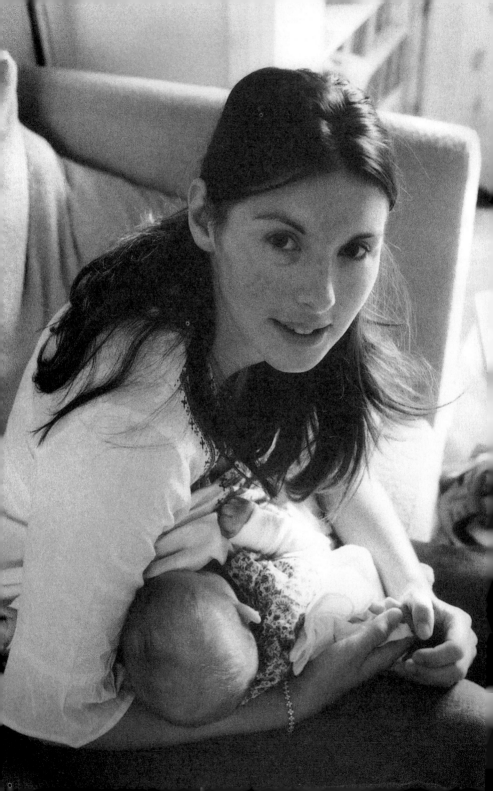

but you really can tell, especially the cries for tiredness and hunger. It's all a matter of getting to know your baby and believing in yourself!

I felt that we were quite lucky with Poppy, as after only three months she had started to sleep through the night with her last full feed at 7:00 pm and her next at about 7:00 am. I am not sure why she was so easy in that way. By this time I found breastfeeding to be a wonderful, exciting and bonding experience. It lasted for about six (mostly) blissful months. So it was with great joy and anticipation that I looked forward to breastfeeding our second baby. Little did I know that this experience was going to be totally different and one that I hope won't put me off breastfeeding any other babies we might be lucky enough to have in the future.

I don't want to put *you* off (if you are planning to breastfeed for the first time) but I feel I should tell you about my bad time, as it is all part of the experience (and I had no idea this could happen).

I was eight months pregnant with Daisy when we went to celebrate Poppy's first birthday with our NCT class. Being the first mum out of our group to get preggers for a second time, I was a source of fascination to all the girls. My friend Sarah asked what I was most looking forward to about becoming a mum for the second time and I said . . . breastfeeding four months down the line!

When Daisy was born a month later, she was given straight to me, as Poppy had been, but instead of having difficulty latching on she fed straightaway and with vigor for at least an hour. I was chuffed that I'd gotten past the first hurdle – done and dusted, or so I thought.

Daisy seemed to latch on well but she would break off after only a couple of minutes. I assumed it was because she wasn't hungry, as it seemed to be happening all the time. I would continually try to get her on the breast, arranging her time and time again so that she would sit on there happily, but no matter what I did, her latch was weak and I often found myself hunched over trying to fit my nipple into her mouth (which I knew was incorrect and would only cause me pain).

After about two weeks I had managed to get used to it, but I knew that something wasn't right. It was on one of my midwife's visits that I decided to discuss this matter with her. I felt a little foolish, as I assumed she would think that by now I had it all figured out, since Daisy had gained a really good daily weight, so what was wrong? The midwife I had was quite vague, and after letting her see how I was feeding she said that there was nothing wrong with Daisy or the technique with which I was feeding her. I was still totally unconvinced. When I looked at Daisy a little closer it looked like there might be a problem with her tongue. We never did get to the bottom of it, but one day she suddenly latched on properly and then she was off!

Within days of my midwife's visit I awoke one morning to find that my left breast was burning hot and covered with red blotchy marks starting from my armpit and spreading down toward my nipple. I had never felt anything like it before and could only assume that I had developed the dreaded mastitis. I could not believe that I had managed to avoid it with Poppy and now it had caught up with me!

It was so painful that if I touched it I felt sick. I should have known that it was coming, as the day before I had started getting flu-like symptoms and had assumed that I was just run-down and tired. But apparently this was a sign that mastitis was setting in. When I woke up the flu-like symptoms had worsened and I was dripping with sweat and shivering under the duvet. I couldn't bear anyone touching me. This was going to be impossible, as I was on my own looking after Poppy and Daisy. And of course the first thing that Poppy wanted in the morning was a huge cuddle and the first thing Daisy wanted was my inflamed boob . . . you must be joking, girls.

I couldn't believe that my body could react so badly to a simple blocked milk duct. The first thing that I knew would ease the pain was a warm bath. Submerged in the water I could feel the pain ease but I knew that this was only a temporary solution – sooner or later I would have to get out!

With the knowledge that the best thing to do with mastitis is to allow your baby to feed off the breast till it was empty (I know, it seemed crazy to me too) I thought I was going to be letting myself in for torture. But the reason that you have to continue feeding is to drain the milk away, otherwise it will lead to a build-up and eventually an abscess – this I did not want. I also tried to do a bit of hand expressing, especially around the tender areas. It seemed to ease the pain for about half an hour, then my breast would harden and inflame again – it was so tiring, especially as I was trying to look after Poppy too. Four hours after getting up that day, I was weeping into the sofa cushions, unable to do anything. The flu symptoms, coupled with my extreme tiredness, had made

me a wreck. On my own and alone (Jamie was at work)
I felt the lowest I had felt since I had given birth to Poppy.

I then tried a classic remedy that my health visitor had
suggested – cabbage leaves! With both babies set down for a
nap I took out two fat green leaves from the fridge and placed
them in my bra – hmm, that was one way to boost a cleavage!
Then I lay out in the sun to try and get warm, even though
I was burning up already. I really don't think the cabbage
leaves did anything, but the fact that they were ice-cold was
a relief in itself. Plus, I don't think that I was beginning to
smell that good. Later that afternoon my bra was emulating
a scent that resembled smelly socks and rotting veg! Yuk,
no thanks! I then decided to use special gel-filled breast pads,
bought when I was pregnant with Poppy, which you could
either stick in the fridge or boil up in a saucepan to make cold
or warm compresses. I decided on the latter and found that
to be quite a relief. Daisy was still feeding off both breasts but
nothing seemed to help.

By late afternoon I couldn't take it any more. I felt as if I had
tropical fever and I didn't look much better either. I will never
forget how I was feeling in the picture opposite. I was slumped
over Poppy's high chair trying to feed her, while holding Daisy
at the same time. My cheeks were burning red and my face
was puffy from crying and, for some reason, I had decided that
it would be a good idea to cut my bangs (à la Catherine Zeta-
Jones). You can't really see from the picture, but my hair
looked dreadful – a cross between Humpty Dumpty and a
bowl cut! Very wrong – I would advise you never to do drastic
things with your hair while high on hormones!

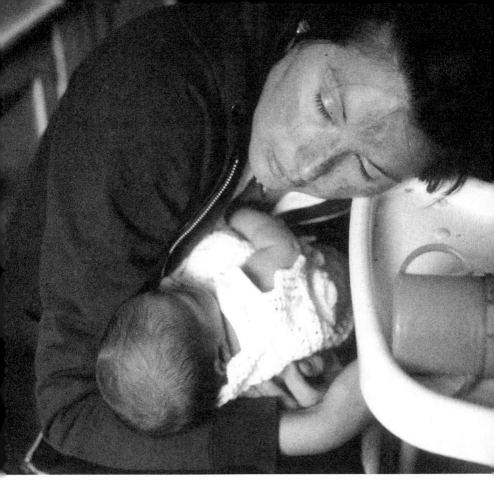

So with me in this state, Jamie decided enough of the herbal remedies – it was time to call the doctor. It was such a relief to see someone medical. I had begun to think that maybe it wasn't mastitis after all but something more sinister! After a quick examination, the doctor confirmed it was mastitis and a course of antibiotics was prescribed. I couldn't get down to the late-night pharmacist quick enough. It was amazing – within one day I was back to my normal self. My breast no longer had the red, splayed blotches all over it and my flu-like symptoms had completely disappeared.

I was so relieved I could now carry on breastfeeding without any pain and discomfort. Four happy days passed until the fifth when I woke in the morning to find that I had those all-too-familiar feelings of pain and soreness in my body, but this time it was the other boob that had the red blotches and the nagging aches. I couldn't believe it. I was still on the antibiotics – how could this be? After a quick visit to my doctor he decided that I should be put on to slightly stronger medication. Again, within hours I was back to my normal self. I hoped that I had beaten it but it was not to be. Five months down the line and I had battled through seven hideous bouts of mastitis – it was an ongoing nightmare.

Each time I was struck down I would read up about it, determined to get to the bottom of why this was happening. After all, it was threatening my decision to carry on, although I was determined to try and see it through, as I wanted to feed Daisy for as long as I had fed Poppy. It was really getting me down. I ended up visiting three different doctors, who each gave me different opinions. Two of them suggested that I give up and start bottle feeding and the other suggested that I feed Daisy through the pain as it would help. I was so confused. I was dying to pack it in, to feed her from a bottle, but that would have left me feeling guilty and I was also driven with a desire to beat it. On the other hand, I was fed up with plying my body with endless antibiotics – what the hell were they doing to my insides?

During one of my reading-up sessions I discovered that

sometimes your baby can pass bacteria to you through your nipple, and each time she feeds she is simply putting it back into your body, which results in mastitis. Armed with this knowledge, I confronted my doctor and, under my instruction, he analyzed a sample of my breast milk to see if it contained any bacteria. I felt like Miss Marple! Alas, no bacteria were found. I was so disappointed, as I really wanted to discover what was causing it. Finally, I decided that enough was enough. I was going to stop breastfeeding – I had managed for five and a half months. If only it was that simple . . . Daisy didn't want the bottle; she wanted the boob. Let the next battle commence!

As I mentioned earlier, Pops' transition from breast to bottle was not an easy one, but if I had known how hard it was going to be with Daisy I never would have complained with the Popster! I persevered with Daisy for many weeks but in the end I decided the best thing would be to introduce someone completely new into Daisy's life to try and get her off the breast. And that someone came in the shape of a maternity nurse called Barbara – my lifesaver.

By this point I was feeling extremely emotional, tired, guilty and worn down, and she was just fantastic. I booked her to come over every day for a week but I honestly didn't have all that much faith. Being a mum twice over made me feel that I should have known what to expect by now and how to cope, but one thing that I've learned is that all babies are not the same and each experience is completely different. I never would have thought that with my second child I would have to call in extra help for what would be deemed as a very simple mummy task! Like a miracle, Barbara had Daisy sucking contentedly on her first bottle of formula on day two!

This whole episode made me realize that I shouldn't feel guilty about calling on other people for help. I really wanted to achieve everything with my two girls and cope with the rough stuff without having to rely on outside help, but it was such a relief to step aside and let go for a minute. After seven rounds of mastitis I would have let Mr. Blobby in to help me, but thank God for Barbara!

I MUST, I MUST . . . DO MY PELVIC FLOORS!

Now if you are anything like me (and, for your sake, let's hope not!), you will join a gym with all the enthusiasm of an Olympic runner and then quite happily pay your membership every month and then, quite happily, NEVER go! It was only after having Poppy that I realized maybe it was time to stop making excuses and get my bum down to the gym, although my GP did tell me that if I hadn't been a big exerciser before I became pregnant then I didn't really have to become superfit overnight. I am by no means a lazy person and I think that I am actually quite fit, but while I was pregnant I considered climbing the stairs to our flat with seven bags of groceries my weekly workout. And that cleaning and scrubbing were my new calisthenics!

The morning after I had given birth to Poppy, I was basking in brand-new motherhood. Various hospital staff would wander in to check on us, and I felt totally pampered until one lady (lovely as she was) came in to discuss the different exercises that I should be doing once I got home. She handed me a leaflet with little pictures of a woman in an assortment of exercise positions – one with her leg cocked in the air and one with her pelvis lifted to the sky. The mere thought of cocking my legs anywhere right now was inconceivable but the lady assured me that this valuable workout would reduce my tummy size and tighten my muscles so that I would heal. Well, that's all well and good, but my promise to do pelvic floors was very short lived. To this day I have probably only done about a hundred of them since having both babies . . . However, if you think you can get away without doing them, like me, then read on to hear about the consequences!

I am now unable to EVER bounce on a trampoline. I tried it last Christmas when Anna, my sister-in-law, bought one for her little boys. I threw myself on to it, very excitedly, only to find myself "leaking" on to my pants. Very embarrassing and extremely uncomfortable! Well, I thought that as I wasn't going to be trampolining every day it wouldn't matter, but I soon realized that a whole range of daily activities would have me peeing left, right and center! There was one classic moment when Jamie and I were hosting a party to celebrate him receiving his MBE (Member of the British Empire, from the Queen). I love a good boogie, so once the disco was in full swing, I let myself go. As my dancing partner for the night, a friend named Asa, flung me in the air, my pelvics failed me and within minutes I was shamefully walking home to change . . . ! So the moral of the story is, you must DO YOUR PELVIC FLOORS! It's so worth the effort in the end.

BABY YOGA AND EXERCISE

After a couple of months as a new mum to Poppy, I decided
that I wanted to get out and do something a little different. I
wanted to stop feeling so damn tired all the time and figured
that exercise would be the best way to do this. I loved the idea
of doing a baby yoga class, as it would be something that Poppy
and I could do together. I came across a local yoga center called
Tri Yoga which was running a class called "Mummy and Me" –
this involved relaxing yoga for the mums and then music,
movement and dancing with your baby. I loved going along
and really looked forward to Tuesday mornings. Getting my
tracksuit bottoms on, I felt like I was part of the world once
more, and Poppy loved the dancing bit when we would waltz
around the room to the Beatles. It was our weekly treat.

Unfortunately, I was unable to take many classes, as I
had to stop going once I found out that I was pregnant
again. From then on, Tuesday mornings never had quite
the same appeal! When Daisy was born I started going to
the classes again, with both the girls and my sister in tow. It
turned out to be a bad idea though, since Poppy wanted to
run around and Lisa couldn't hold her yoga poses while
trying to hold Poppy still at the same time! After a couple of
weeks we gave up. I do find that this sort of thing happens
at most social gatherings or events now, and I have to have
eyes in the back of my head to keep tabs on both the girls.

After the yoga sessions had stopped I decided that the only
way to get fit was to work out properly. It was quite hard to find
time during the day, so I decided to be extravagant and hired a

personal trainer who specialized in postnatal exercise. This was perfect for me, as Daisy was still only about eight weeks old and I wanted to shift the paunch which I had developed.

Fiona was an excellent trainer. She came to the house once a week and boy did she make me work! I would dread the sessions and think of a million excuses the night before that might sound plausible to get me out of doing them. But each time I did them I felt fabulous afterward – energized, revitalized and a teeny bit slimmer. Soon, though, Fiona became pregnant and our sessions had to come to an end; but not before she dragged me around Hampstead Heath on our weekly jogs when she was six months pregnant! I was often mistaken for her trainer as she pounded through the woods with me flagging behind, shouting various expletives and waving my arms around to ease the ever-growing stitch in my side!

Anyway, it has taken me up until now to have the motivation to go to the gym on a more regular basis. Both Poppy and Daisy have little membership cards and have been to the gym more times than me! A couple of weeks ago I persuaded my friend Amy, who is also a mum of two, to get down to the gym. Our plan is to push each other, knowing that when we drop the girls off at nursery school on Monday, Wednesday and Friday mornings, we are to be decked out in our tracksuits and ready for action. Woe betide one of us if we dare turn up in jeans professing to be too tired!

CHAPTER SIX

Baby – The First Three Months

I had absolutely NO idea just how much our lives would change when Poppy was born, and then again with Daisy, but I was about to find out.

I remember that first night in the hospital with Poppy beside me in her bassinet. It was . . . well, actually there are no words to describe just how truly wonderful it was. It's quite hard to recapture those feelings as it is such a unique time. Poppy was born at 3:08 in the afternoon and I can recall that the rest of the afternoon went by in a haze. I was propped up in my bed with Jamie nearby and Poppy in my arms in her big blanket. We had a stream of visitors wishing us well – my mum and sisters, and Jamie's parents and sister. It was like being in a dream and one that I hoped I wouldn't have to wake up from! When everyone had left and it was just the three of us it dawned on me that we were now a mummy and a daddy and everything was going to be different.

Jamie had gone home, as I was starving and he was worried that honey on toast was not enough after all the hard work I had just put in. I didn't have the heart to tell him that I had already consumed a Mars Bar and half a Kit Kat, so as he zoomed off home to whip up something fantastic and chef-like for me, I lay facing Poppy's little plastic cot and marveled at just how adorable she was. I must have fallen asleep, as the next thing I knew Poppy wasn't in her cot and instead I was staring at a huge bowl of Jamie's homemade Pukkola (it's like luxury muesli). I panicked and rang the bell for the midwife. Apparently Poppy had woken up crying and the midwives had managed to settle her. Relieved, I cradled her in my arms and dug into the first decent meal I had had in three days, and it was great.

The next day I was excited to get home and practically begged my obstetrician to release me as early as possible! Poppy and I hastily had all our final examinations while Jamie signed all the paperwork.

POST-PARTUM BLEEDING . . . SOME THINGS YOU SHOULD KNOW

This is probably the best place to mention post-partum bleeding. I don't want to scare anybody, but if my labor story hasn't put you off yet then let me try with the bit that is often left out of your prenatal class discussions! You may have to have stitches after a vaginal delivery, which will lead to a bit of bleeding and, if you're unlucky (like me) these could be second-degree stitches which leave you with ongoing pain way after everyone has gone home, the last cupcake has been eaten and your baby is snuggled up in a basket. Whether you have a normal delivery or a caesarean, you will also have normal vaginal bleeding for anything up to a few weeks.

As if it isn't bad enough in the days after giving birth that you're not only extremely exhausted and your nipples look and feel like the top of Mount Etna right after an eruption; your (how shall I put it?) swollen lower regions are extremely tender as well.

I just did not realize:

* How much I would bleed after having a baby. I think that I got through three brick-shaped maternity pads a day (I did wonder, before I went into the hospital, why I just couldn't use the normal-sized sanitary pads with wings – I soon found out!).
* How sore I would feel. So much so that I was given three bottles of painkillers when I was discharged from the hospital.
* How harrowing my first . . . poo might be! After delivering Poppy I think I was constipated for five days because I was so afraid that if I did go, everything else might go as well (if you know what I mean). Of course, so I can put your mind at ease, I did eventually go and nothing bad happened. In fact, it was just like normal – even if I was left shaking afterward!

Apart from the painkillers that I was given by the hospital, I found a "vaginal ice pack" at home that I'd bought but didn't think I'd ever use. It's a gel-filled pack in the shape of a pad so that you can fit it in your underwear. You can stick it in the fridge to cool it down first then when you wear it the pain is soothed and numbed. One of these comes highly recommended by me; although Jamie wasn't too impressed when he saw me in some lovely underwear padded out with a gel-pack in my pants and an equally dodgy-looking one in each bra cup – the best contraception money can buy!

Although it all sounds awful, this discomfort is only temporary. And you must keep thinking that it's worth it, because after all you will have the most precious and beautiful baby to take your mind off it. The bleeding lasts for around two weeks, the stitches will fall out and soon you'll start to feel like your old self again. And that's when you might very well get . . . hemorrhoids!

WHAT HAPPENS NEXT?

When I left the hospital I was given a brown envelope and on the front it said that a midwife would visit me the next day. In Britain, your local community midwife will have been told about you and the baby. You don't need to worry about contacting anyone yourself. They will just turn up to see you at some point the next day. I found that bit really helpful as it was a chance to chat with someone who knew what they were doing, and to find out the baby's weight.

First of all she checks you over if you've had stitches or a caesarean – she'll check your wound and ask how you feel. Then she'll ask if you've gone to the bathroom properly yet and about your blood loss. Sometimes your midwife will ask you to demonstrate your breastfeeding technique and she'll check your nipples if you want her to, to make sure they're not cracked or sore. In Britain, the midwife will continue to visit you every day for about ten days but if you want her to continue coming then she will. Or, if you feel that you have everything under control, she will only come for a few days and then leave her number with you for emergencies. Every time she visits she will ask for your notes which you should always have on hand. She will leave you with a "red book" which has all the baby's notes in it. She will fill it out for you and then leave it with you. You'll also be given a card to register the baby with a pediatrician and you must do this during the first week if you can.

Then I had a visit from the health visitor – I wasn't quite sure what her role was. I was quite nervous, as I thought she might judge my parenting skills and analyze me for postpartum depression to see if I'd been crying too much. But don't be daunted by them, as they are there to help you out as well – you can use them as a first line of defense if you have any worries, instead of calling your GP all the time. It's good to have someone like this on the end of a phone – they will probably leave you their mobile phone number. I used to call mine every couple of months to ask about rashes, or breast to bottle feeding. General things. I would look these things up in books, but it was nice to have someone at the end of the phone as well.

Like most brand-new mums and dads, leaving the hospital is a really exciting moment but mine was extremely nerve-wracking as well, because outside Queen Charlotte's Hospital there were about 30 photographers, like animals awaiting their prey. But as we emerged I, for once, didn't feel shy but completely proud to show off our Poppy. I suddenly felt a huge surge of confidence – maybe it was because I was now a mummy and I had to be responsible and grown up. I had a little person who was totally dependent on me; I was in charge; I was her protector. It felt great.

Well, I thought I was in charge but little Pops had other ideas! No sooner had I carried her over the threshold in her ultra-cute fluffy bunny suit than she promptly deposited all her milk on my lap and gave the biggest burp I had ever heard! I immediately turned to my mum and started to panic, wondering if she was all right. I thought she might choke – thank goodness Mum was there. I REALLY didn't have a clue about what I was doing! Little things like not knowing how to do up the snaps on a sleeper suddenly seem like huge problems, but you soon learn. There are so many things to worry about; so many unanswered questions, but you just get on with it as you go along. I remember worrying about the right room temperature for the baby, or what she should be wearing – how do you know that she's not overheating in what you've dressed her in for bed?

To give me some support and to show me the ropes, I had arranged with Mum that she would stay with us for a week. It was lovely to have her there because it felt so reassuring. I knew that she wouldn't have had it any other way. Plus, Jamie now had someone there who would really appreciate his cooking and his love of a good glass of vino at the end of a long day!

It was like being a little girl again. Mum looked after me amazingly; I was totally spoiled and it was just what I needed! For the first few days, Poppy would sleep all day. I couldn't understand it and even called my midwife to ask if this was normal! She laughed and said, "For goodness sake, make use of it now as it won't last long!" She was right, of course!

Mum tried to persuade me to nap at the same time as Poppy in order to store my energy for the long night ahead, but all I wanted to do was either cuddle Pops or put about 10 loads of washing on while cleaning and tidying the kitchen. Not to mention the ironing – all of which my mum insisted on banning while she was there.

Mum also showed us how to change a diaper on our first day. Jamie naturally took to it like a duck to water, whereas I took a while longer. I don't know why, as changing a diaper now is second nature. Bathing Poppy was another job which we were both clueless about, but, again, it's a really easy task and very enjoyable too. On day three I decided to take matters into my own hands and bathe Poppy all by myself. I was worried that I would become too reliant on Mum and go utterly to pieces when she left. So, armed with all the necessary equipment, I nervously took Poppy up to the nursery. I don't really know what I was afraid of, but as Mum and Jamie sat downstairs with their glasses of red wine, pretending not to listen intently, I undressed Poppy. She immediately started crying. I knew that I should have closed the window first – it was obviously too cold for her. I quickly placed her in her little sink (which she had practically outgrown by this time and she was only two days old) and this sent her into even more of a tearful frenzy. Oh God – this didn't happen when Jamie did it. I didn't know how to stop the crying so I whipped her out and tried to cuddle her, but by now she was ticked off. I think she could tell that it was Mummy's first time and so she let rip with all the strength she could muster and, just for good measure, as I fumbled

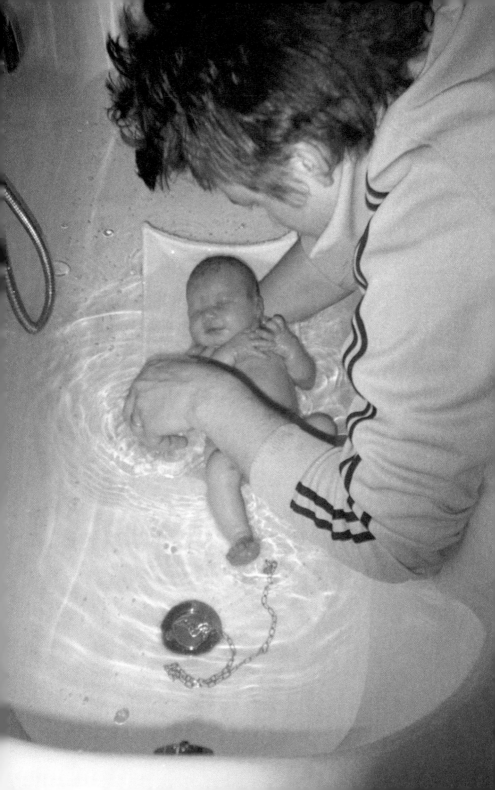

with getting her onesie on (I was all hot and panicky by this stage) she peed all over my lap. This was a disaster. I'm just no good at it, I thought. Soaking wet, sweating and red-faced, I came downstairs with Poppy now happy and smelling delicious. I must have looked quite the picture but even if I did my two best friends simply said, "Well done, you did brilliantly!" I don't think I will ever forget just how proud of myself I felt then.

OUR FIRST TRIP OUT AS A FAMILY

I remember the first time Jamie and I ventured out of the house with Pops very vividly. It was exactly five days after she was born and I was raring to get out and about into the fresh air (well, as fresh as air can get in north London) and show off our little bundle to the world!

It was a gorgeous spring morning. I was so excited about getting out of the house that I woke up even earlier than Poppy and was in the shower marveling at how much my tummy had shrunk (but it was still bloody huge – all rippling, pudgy and wobbly!) compared to five days ago. I thought I was looking pretty good for a girl who had just given birth. And what couldn't be shoved neatly into my button-fly jeans wasn't worth worrying about anyway.

So, with me all suited and baseball-booted and ready to go, there was just the simple task of getting Pops ready and the slightly harder task of getting Jamie out of bed.

After an hour of cajoling Jamie and waiting for Poppy to wake up, my enthusiasm and energy were seriously waning.

I couldn't think why I had been so excited; after all, our first outing was to Borough Market (a Saturday morning food market which Jamie shops at for all the dream produce he uses to make our usual mammoth weekend feasts). I had never really loved going. I went a few times when I was pregnant, but when it's –5 degrees early on a January morning, nothing, not even a bacon roll made with fresh organic meat from Prince Charles' estate, could lift my spirits! It just wasn't my thing. Had we gotten up early to browse through my favorite clothing store, well, now you're talking, pregnant or not!

Obviously there was a slight bone of contention between Jamie and me about where our first outing with Poppy would be to. Borough Market is *his* passion and he really wanted to show Poppy off to his friends there. I would have preferred a trip to the shops or a walk in the local park. I do have to admit, though, that on some occasions I have really enjoyed wandering around Borough Market, sampling all the wonderful produce (especially the cake stalls – that's one passion I keep to myself!). The sights, the smells, the characters – it's all there on a Saturday morning, but then so is my steaming cappuccino, our squashy sofa and a roaring fire at home.

Nowadays, Jamie takes both our girls to Borough Market most Saturday mornings. For me it's a chance to actually eat my breakfast in total peace without little feet and hands climbing all over me and without food being smeared on the floor. And for Jamie, crazy though I think he is, his treat after a whole week at work is to take his little girls, wrapped up in their coats and bundled into the car, to the market. The stories I hear when they get home are fantastic. Both girls always come running in with samples that the market has to offer down the front of their clothes, but they're so happy. Poppy launches into a story about everything that's happened, from drinking strawberry milkshakes, to dancing with the resident old lady busker, to being serenaded by the wonderful veg man who by night is a fantastic soprano singer (he even sang at Poppy's christening!). So our weekends usually start with everyone contented and happy.

Well, that is now, but back then Poppy had no idea while I got her dressed that morning that she was about to visit somewhere that her dad would end up taking her to every week! Mum helped me figure out the appropriate outfit for Poppy to be seen in on her first official public appearance! I remember it well – it was a vibrant blue onesie with "100% PERFECT" emblazoned across it, and I thought she looked adorable. Naturally, while Jamie was still in bed, I had packed and repacked her diaper bag and it was propped up against the door ready to go. Yes, you've guessed it, turn the page to see another mammoth list showing exactly what we took out with us that day. . . . I'm not sure how I fitted it all in!

So there you have it. One extremely heavy bag to carry around. And we used absolutely none of it. Now, after three years of motherhood, I've managed to keep things to the bare minimum when going on a short journey (a little makeup bag with two diapers, a couple of diaper disposal bags, a bag of the oh-SO-essential baby wipes, two burping clothes and two

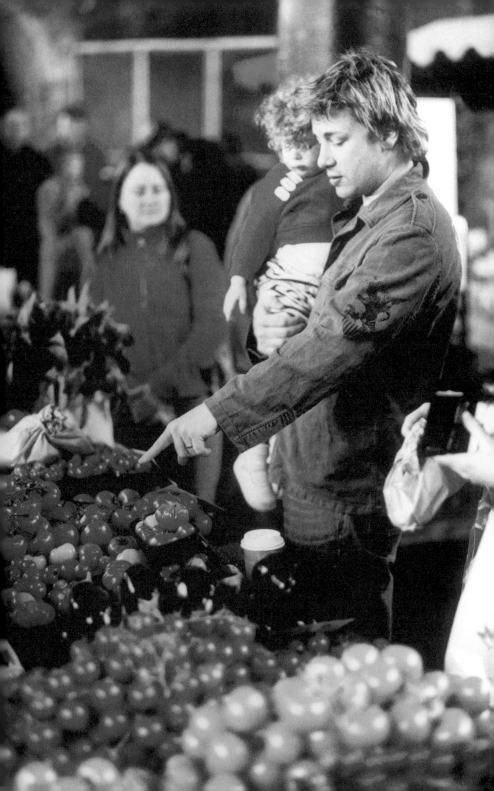

Poppy's Change Bag

- 3 white babygrows in case of milk spillage, poo leakage or any other orifice explosion!

- 4 white muslins – 2 for her to snuggle against and 2 for the reason the fantastic muzzi was invented (mopping up!)

- 2 bibs – not that I ever actually used them but that's what it advised in my baby mag!

- 10 nappies (what was I thinking? She wasn't even on solids yet ... now that's when 10 nappies come in handy!)

- 1 box of scented nappy sacks
- 1 bag of pleated cotton wool
- 1 bottle of warmed water in a bottle for wiping her little bum
- 4 rattles and various cuddly toys, plus a little wind-up musical toy (all these things went completely over her head, literally, as she was asleep for the whole 4-hour trip!)
- 4 breast pads for me
- 2 of the biggest maternity pads you have ever seen
- 1 pot of Sudocrem
- 1 cellular blanket

And finally, a little woolly hat, in case we lost the one she was wearing!

(I realize that some of these terms might be confusing! Nappies, as I'm sure you know, are diapers. Muslins—muzzis for short—are just little burping cloths. Sudacrem is a brand of diaper-rash ointment. And a cellular blanket is the sort of soft, holey blanket they give you in the hospital when the baby is born.)

packets of raisins!). On the other hand, though, both my daughters seem to pack a suitcase each when leaving the house to go shopping. I mean, how could they bear to be separated from half the contents of their toy box for one hour? I wonder where they get it from!

So, back to Poppy at five days old . . . We were about to set off to the market but there was just the one small matter of which carriage we should take. Stupidly, we hadn't bothered to do a little test run with either of them before Pops was born, so half of the parts were still in the box and neither of us had a clue how to erect them! So, in true Jamie style, he chucked all the pieces for one of the carriages in the trunk of the car and hoped that it would sort itself out at the other end. Of course, on arrival, the scene was entitled "How Many People Does It Take to Put Together a Carriage?" Why on earth does all baby equipment have to be made so DAMN hard to assemble? How many times have I stood in the pouring rain struggling with an irate toddler and mini toddler while trying to clip two simple pieces of plastic together to make a seat harness? Why is it always such a palaver? And why is it that with the double-buggy I find myself thrashing it around to open it up and only when I have chipped a nail, snagged my thumb and made myself bleed will it relent and open up? I then find myself having to jump down on it to click it into place. If my eldest daughter were to suddenly come out with an extremely rude expletive, I won't blame myself or Jamie, but the manufacturers who sell this awkward, complicated baby gear . . . well, I feel a lot better now I've got that off my chest! But just to really twist the knife, here are my top five irritations about baby equipment. It might help you to remain calm if you find yourself in the same position:

- ✢ **Car seats** – don't even go there if your child has a bulky winter coat on and is buckerooing out of the seat in a temper at the same time . . . WHY, WHY, WHY aren't the straps longer and less fiddly?
- ✢ **Buggies** – I don't care which make or model they are, but when you are trying to open them and they are stiff, it's a nightmare.
- ✢ **Toys** – I know it's for safety reasons but why on earth do toys come packaged like they are Fort Knox? The twisted wire and hard plastic is infuriating!
- ✢ **Baby carriers** – all fab in theory, but try and grapple with one when you and the baby have both got winter coats on, you're sweating, the baby is hysterical and you can't work out your Strap A from your Strap B – a nightmare!
- ✢ **Buggy boards** – again, very practical and clever but it's a near impossibility to erect them. We have been through three of them as they either broke by themselves or by me in a temper! My sister and I attempted to attach the first one to the buggy, then one of our contractors did the second one for me and then the third (yes, the third!) I asked Jamie to do, but that one has fallen by the wayside, so I am OVER them!

Anyway, that was quite a big digression, but after just 35 minutes of baby carriage assembly Jamie, Mum and I were ready to go. Pops had given up on the useless threesome and fallen asleep, and for the first time we placed her car seat on to her pram (we had one of those travel systems where the car seat clicks on to the pram). Wow, this felt great, and didn't she look adorable?! There was a little bit of a struggle between the three of us over who was to push her but Jamie got the long straw. He pushed her through the market – he couldn't hide his pride – and with me clutching on to one of the handles and my mum continually fussing with the blanket we must have looked like the perfect family!

That weekend I was determined to use every baby accessory and bit of equipment that I owned. After a wonderful lunch munching on all our delicious goods that we had bought from the market, we decided on an afternoon stroll but this time I wanted to carry Poppy in her baby sling. Now that really was a treat – she felt so cozy and warm against me. Apart from worrying that I might be suffocating her, the whole experience was brilliant (and it didn't take us four hours to get out of the house like it had that morning!).

On the Sunday we decided to take a stroll around Hampstead Heath. Funny really, we had lived in Hampstead for three years and never really used the Heath, and now we have our babies that's all we ever do! But this time I thought that instead of the baby sling or our Mamas and Papas three-in-one system we would use the Adventurer pram (something that we were coerced and seduced into buying, on the promise that we could push the buggy through all kinds of muddy terrain and rocky mountain (i.e. the Heath!) with ease and sophistication). I think that after two long hours of nursery shopping on a Saturday afternoon, Jamie was hallucinating and imagined he was shopping for an episode of *Top Gear*!

Not only could we barely fit this super pram in the house, we also couldn't collapse it . . . naturally! But, again, after much swearing and sweating, the Adventurer was ready to go. It was so wide and heavy that it didn't even fit down the narrow streets of Hampstead. This meant that we ended up running down the hill throwing everyone else out of our path. It was like taking a Great Dane for a walk, not a 7 lb. 14 oz. baby for a stroll. There was no time to stop and chat to any well wishers – not even Jamie had the strength to hold her back; this pram had a mind of its own and it was going to destroy everything and everyone in its path. To be fair to the pram, it was on an adventure (that was its name, after all), but unfortunately not with this family, so no sooner had we pushed Poppy back up the hill to home, than we threw it in the cupboard and promptly gave it to a lovely pregnant friend of ours (but failed to mention the demonic qualities that it possessed!).

So, our road test was complete. After checking the scores we decided that for the time being, the baby sling was our safest and easiest mode of transportation. It also meant that I could harness Poppy into it in the comfort and safety of our own home, without the paparazzi getting sneaky shots of me with my plumber butt in the air desperately trying to erect the pram in the street.

ON OUR OWN . . .

And so our first week together drew to a close. Mum asked me if I wanted her to stay a bit longer. As much as I did, I knew that it was time for her to go. Jamie was starting to go back to work again and I wanted to experience all I could without her before he went. The afternoon Mum left, I was very emotional. I didn't realize the impact that it would have on me when she finally got into her taxi. She put on her dark glasses – she always does this when she doesn't want to show us she's crying (doesn't take a genius to realize where I get it from!).

This was it. We were really on our own now. I had Jamie there with me for a bit longer, but I was quite nervous about him going back to work, as I would then be completely on my own with Poppy for the first time. However, being alone is the jolt you need in order to get on with being a mum. And it's actually never as frightening as you might imagine; you finally realize that, "Yes, I can do this," and, "It's going to be okay." Goodness knows what it must be like for women who have twins or triplets – much respect to you if you are one of them! And if you're a single mum, or dad, then the biggest admiration to you. It was hard enough with two of us, and I can't think what it would have been like to tackle it alone.

With Mum gone, I didn't really know what to do first. It was about the time for Poppy's bath, so I thought, "Here we go." Only half an hour later I came down with Poppy. I was as red as could be with my boobs on display and my tracksuit (make that Jamie's) halfway down my butt. Pops, however, was in her little pink baby suit and she smelled divine again! And there, laid out on our little coffee table in the sitting room was a beautiful dinner specially prepared by my husband! I promptly burst into tears and of course that got Pops going too. Then I couldn't stop crying – the tears just kept flowing and flowing, in between some laughter. Even Poppy got bored after an hour and decided that enough was enough. She was ready for her bouncy chair and a little bit of shut-eye. "Mum's just weird," she was probably thinking and, to be honest, I was beginning to think that I was as well. I actually started to believe that I had developed postnatal depression as I wept for hours. What made it worse was that I was watching *Titanic* – of all films. I had seen it before and had not shed a single tear but now I was crying enough water to sink the *Titanic* myself!

The emotions that had been pent up for the last $9^{1}/_{2}$ months had finally come to a head. I didn't realize just how many tears I had stored up. And do you know what, those tears never stop! Sometimes there is absolutely no reason for them, so it's not always best to question them; better to let them flow and then cheer yourself up by going shopping! Jamie was brilliant and he helped me to laugh through the tears or sometimes surprised me by bringing home a small present.

The next few weeks all seemed to roll into one. I never really knew what day it was, as weekends became weekdays and Poppy's naps became my new official bedtimes – it was the only way to try and beat the relentless fatigue that would sweep over me as I trudged through the day. I know that this is beginning to sound like hell, but, on the upside, Poppy would do something new and wonderful every day. These little things would obliterate all our tiredness and make us extremely happy.

I had really started to establish some sort of routine by about week two. I know that sounds a little military and strict for a baby so young, but it was a way of getting some order back into our lives after they had been turned upside down and inside out, back to front and around the bend. So anything that made things structured was all right with us! I had already established a sort of breastfeeding routine every four hours, but of course this was not at all possible at the beginning as Poppy spent all her days asleep and I really didn't want to wake her just to stick to a timetable! But, as time went on, she was more awake during the day and it made sense for me to try and set out a routine that would help both of us.

I realized straight off that you have to be extremely organized as a mum. It's the only way I was able to get on top of everything and manage to get all my jobs done as well. So, first thing in the morning I would even do simple things like getting Poppy's pajamas, diaper and towel out next to her changing mat in our bathroom so it was all ready for the nighttime bath. This made it so much easier than running around gathering everything while an already fractious Poppy lay waiting to be dressed after her bath. Simple things like drawing the curtains and getting her little crib ready in our bedroom, setting the temperature and nightlight, for example, would all be done before her bath. It made me feel far more relaxed and ahead of myself, which, quite frankly, I think you need when you have such a precious newborn to care for.

I had already established our little routine when I came across *The Contented Little Baby Book*. Now, I had heard these five words many times before – they were first bandied around our prenatal class with much discussion. Everyone seemed to get very heated and opinionated about this book. Some loved the idea behind it, some hated it and others just seemed too scared to even give an opinion. I was intrigued by all this. How could a book like this cause so much confrontation? I didn't get to read it until one day when I received a beautiful gift box from a friend, full of fun and useful things to welcome Poppy and to see us through the early stages of parenthood. Between the bottle of vodka and the Baby Einstein videos was this much talked-about book with a little note attached to it saying "This book is essential reading. It allowed us to have our nights back – hurray!" Wow, that sounded like a promise I couldn't pass up.

Naturally and, as expected, we hadn't had a good night's sleep since Pops was born. Of course we couldn't really complain because this was what being a parent was all about, but I had never imagined just how much the lack of sleep would affect us. At first it was all exciting and a real novelty to have us both up and walking around like zombies, but after a while Jamie could no longer get up in the middle of the night just to support me while I breastfed. He had to get up for work in the morning, so then it was just me up at night and I can honestly say sleep deprivation was a shock. I found it very hard to deal with. This *Contented Little Baby Book* seemed to promise so much. As I read it, I couldn't believe that it was possible to be able to get a little baby into an even stricter routine than mine at the tender age of 14 days. I didn't like the sound of this. But as I read on, many of the famous Gina Ford views made sense. However, I felt that her routine at two weeks was far too much for my daughter so I decided to put the book away until I felt it was time to set such a structure. I already had my own little pattern that I had worked out for myself and which I felt was just fine for now.

In the beginning, Poppy used to do all her napping and

sleeping in her bouncy chair, which was fantastic. After her last feed of the day at 7:00 pm, I would gently place her in the chair after she had fallen asleep on my boob. By then she'd be bathed and in her cozy pajamas, ready for bed, but while Jamie and I had our dinner or watched TV she would be right there with us, sometimes lying awake, sometimes deep in sleep with her arms splayed out either side. As the night went on, we found ourselves creeping around the sitting room. We would even talk in whispers so as not to wake her after three or four hours of peace – we had become accustomed to how lovely it felt to have that time to ourselves, knowing that she would soon be waking up and my night would turn into the night shift!

Either way, we would end up staying up late or, more often than not, I would fall asleep on the sofa with Poppy splayed out next to me in her bouncer. This meant that at about one in the morning Jamie would wake me up and insist that I went to bed and we would carry Poppy gently upstairs without waking her – this involved lots of loud whispering from both of us, usually with raised tempers as one of us would, more often than not, make a slight noise going up the stairs. Whoever it was that made the sound which woke Poppy would be the one who would be blamed for anything and everything. Generally it was me who would be blaming Jamie for disturbing our child, and for world hunger for that matter. In that state of tiredness I would tell him off about anything!

This had to stop. It was making me exhausted and we were waking Poppy up unnecessarily. It was ridiculous. I was going to have to get to bed earlier and, more importantly,

I was going to have to get Poppy into her crib at a decent hour so she could get used to having her bath and milk before being settled down. At least this way Jamie and I would be able to eat in complete freedom without worrying that we were going to wake her up. Naturally, this was easier said than done as Jamie didn't get home from work until late, so it was up to me to set up this little routine myself.

The first night I put it into action I remember I had managed to attend one of the prenatal-class gatherings that the other girls had arranged. We were relaxing in Primrose Hill Park with our babies and discussing the usuals when I realized the time. Good God, it was past 5:30 pm. I had to get back! There was bath, boob and bedtime to cram in, and I was running late! It was then, as I mentally stressed out on the way home battling with the traffic, that I realized that this is what life was going to be like if I followed a routine. Keeping time for me had never been a problem before, but now I had a little person to worry about as well, everything seemed to take twice as long . . . funny that! But I had to give it a try. I firmly believed in a routine for children. I would have loved to have been more of a Mediterranean mum, whereby the babies could eat with us into the early hours, supping on leftover glasses of vino and falling asleep past midnight but, unfortunately, we don't live in Italy and weeknight dinners aren't the same when you're on your own and too knackered to cook anyway! So, some sort of a routine would suit me and our lifestyle just fine.

As I said, after studying Gina Ford's book I was shocked. I didn't really understand why it had to be so strict, even down to how much water a breastfeeding mother should drink and at what time of day. But I did appreciate the way she structured the day. It seemed simple and adaptable and something that would suit us, so I dipped in and out of the book, stealing an idea and making it my own and then set about trying to implement it . . . well, easier said than done! As I rushed back home from the park that late afternoon to try out the routine for the first time I was both nervous and excited. After all, this routine could change our lives and maybe, just maybe, Jamie and I would finally get a better night's sleep.

It was really quite basic and went something like this:

I would have to get Poppy up at 7:00 am and give her the first feeding of the day. At around 9:00 am I would put her down for her morning nap for half an hour, then at 10:30 am I would give her her next. After a bit of play or a walk I would put her down for her lunchtime nap at 12:00 pm till 2:15-ish. Then it was up again for her third feed of the day at 2:30 pm, then playtime till 4:00 pm. Then I would take her for a walk, for another little power nap, before taking her home and playing till 5:30-ish. Then she would have a bath. The last feed of the day would be at about 6:00 pm and then bed by 7:00 pm. So that was it. It all sounded so simple. If it all went according to plan then it sounded like a dream.

That first night all started well. I had her bathed and fed by 6:30 pm; however, she fell asleep on my breast, which meant that I was cheating at the routine as I would put her down for the night not being fully awake and aware of her surroundings. If she was to wake up in her new crib all alone, as opposed to being in her bouncer in the front room with

Jamie and me and the TV for company, then it would be a shock. She would then never learn to fall asleep naturally and would rely on my boob forever!

But, quite frankly, it was impossible to work this routine on a baby at such a young age, as she spent most of her time asleep and there was no way that I was going to wake her up! However, the first successful time I put her to sleep in her crib, when she finally settled, I realized how blissful it was to come downstairs and be baby-free for a couple of hours. I felt like me again. I could put the TV on at a higher volume and know that she couldn't hear it as she was snug and secure in her little crib in our bedroom. But, of course, it wasn't long before I would hear her little cries start to build to ear-piercing yells when she realized that she wasn't in her bouncy chair and where was I – guiltily munching on salted cashews and drinking a glass of wine? No! I was back on duty and ready for action. Frantically flicking through my manual, I read that I wasn't to feed Poppy again if she awoke but use other methods to soothe her back to sleep. However, after 45 minutes of constant pacing and rocking I would give in and feed her – it worked instantly and she was soon off to sleep.

It wasn't long before I understood that there were reasons behind all these different rules and tasks set out by the routine. What I hadn't realized was that sometimes Poppy had gas or colic – this may have been due to the fact that I would let her fall asleep on the breast. I'd then put her straight into her crib and not dare to wind her in case she woke up so this was half the problem and explained why she would wake up after only 30 minutes. Other nights I would try and leave her to cry. I know that sounds horrendous and cruel – believe me, I didn't feel remotely good about it – and, in fact, it made me unhappy to the point that Jamie often found me curled up in a heap with tears in my eyes and my head stuck to our bedroom door. Confused and upset, some nights we would find ourselves doing this together and we'd only go downstairs when she was completely zonked out. Although this method was hard, it really did work – especially if I knew that she had fed enough and I had winded her and that she was tired. Only then did I feel strong enough to leave her crying so that she could fall asleep on her own.

The next big step was cutting out nighttime feedings. Obviously in the early stages I fed her when she required it, no matter what time it was, but as I got into the routine and knew that she no longer needed her feed at night I stopped it altogether. It wasn't long after this transition that I woke up to find that it was . . . MORNING! Yeah – it wasn't the middle of the night and I had had a whole night's sleep!

I couldn't get my head around it so woke Jamie up, excited that we had finally managed a whole night without a feed. I felt fantastic and rested. A new woman. When you are up breastfeeding a newborn in the middle of those long nights it doesn't ever seem possible, but now it had happened and I was so happy!

The routine had worked. It hadn't been easy, but I could happily say that my girl was now a truly contented baby. Her morning nap always allowed me to have time to tidy the kitchen and have a bath, get dressed and ready myself to be a mum, and her two-hour-long sleep at lunchtime was a godsend as well. It allowed me to read the papers for the first time in ages, to have lunch (something I hadn't done properly in months) and do a million loads of washing! In fact, I still stick to this routine even now with both the girls, and Poppy is two and a half. I know very well that she has no intention of having her morning nap at 9:00 am on the days when she's not out at nursery, but it fits in with Daisy's routine, so while I have my bath Poppy sits happily in her bed reading or singing, perfectly contented with her own company, whilst I manage to have a bit of me time as well.

Thinking back to this routine lark, it wasn't always easy. There were times when I was just too tired to stick to the rigidity of it. And it would wind Jamie up if I refused to change plans which could potentially muck up the routine, but I would always remind him that if he relished his evenings of coming home to a nice dinner and some cuddle-time on the sofa then we had to stick to the routine. He didn't need much reminding that this scenario was miles better than having to spend his evenings trying to soothe an inconsolable overtired baby for hours on end! And I would find it hard when, for example, I had to wake Poppy at 7:00 am for her first morning feeding having been up with her at 4:00 am so that we were both zonked out, but I was determined to stick with it, not really understanding how it would work now anyway with all her feeding times going out the window.

Sometimes the routine killed me but how can I complain when both our girls go to bed together at 6:30 pm and sleep through till 7:30 the next morning? And they both seem to be happy contented little treasures – well, most of the time!

Certainly, for the first three months there were many sacrifices that had to be made, especially by me, to get things working smoothly. After many weeks of sleepless nights, I soon realized that I would have to be in bed earlier in order to feel somewhat human the next day, so it was with great reluctance that I would wrench myself off the sofa and get into bed by 8:30 pm. Unfortunately, this meant that I wouldn't get to see Jamie some nights because by the time he was home from work I would be tucked up in bed with Poppy sleeping contentedly in her crib beside me.

LAMB CASSEROLE BONK!

You're probably wondering why I'm putting this particular bit of information in the section where Poppy is still only three months old, but read on . . . !

I remember my mum-in-law, Sally, saying that once you got through the first six weeks of your baby's life the rest would become a lot easier and, in a way, she was right, although for me it did take a little longer.

When Poppy reached eight weeks old she was sleeping through the night and I was beginning to feel a little more rested and confident as a mum. I remember one such day when Poppy was being a dream and the day had run unusually smoothly. So much so that I decided to be a little wild and cook Jamie a surprise meal as a treat for us both. He had a rare night off and I really wanted him to come home to a freshly cooked dinner with the smells wafting all around the house. It had been a while since I had done anything like this for him, so I swiftly set about organizing our romantic dinner for two. In an ideal world I would have greeted Jamie at the door with my apron on . . . and nothing else! But this was the two-months-postpartum real world!

First, I had to think of the menu. What on earth was I going to cook? This can be quite hard when it's for Jamie. I had to go simple because I also wanted to make the table look gorgeous and romantic – I decided to try and go all out for one night only (as I wouldn't be doing this again for a while)!

Okay, so it was going to be lamb casserole (no appetizer, let's not overdo it!) with a freshly cooked peach-and-strawberry crumble with custard to follow (his favorite). That would give me enough time to cook it all and still have time to bathe Poppy and have her asleep by 7:00 pm if all went according to plan.

I'm really good at making casseroles – lamb, chicken, vegetable, you name it! Better to be safe than sorry I thought, so that was the reason for choosing it. Crumbles are also one of my specialities, so I was set to go. I have to admit, I couldn't do this every night – it would drive me insane. I am definitely not cut out to be a Stepford Wife just yet!

Anyway, as I whipped up my crumble mix I heard that familiar little cry coming from upstairs. I prayed that perhaps it was one of her murmurs, but the wail to end all wails soon followed. As I dashed upstairs, I wondered if I really would be able to cope with being a perfect wife and a fantastic mother at the same time. This was hard. Clock-watching as I breastfed Poppy, I started to stress. I was never going to get this meal cooked in time – this would be a disaster.

Thank God for Jamie's as-ever appalling timekeeping. For

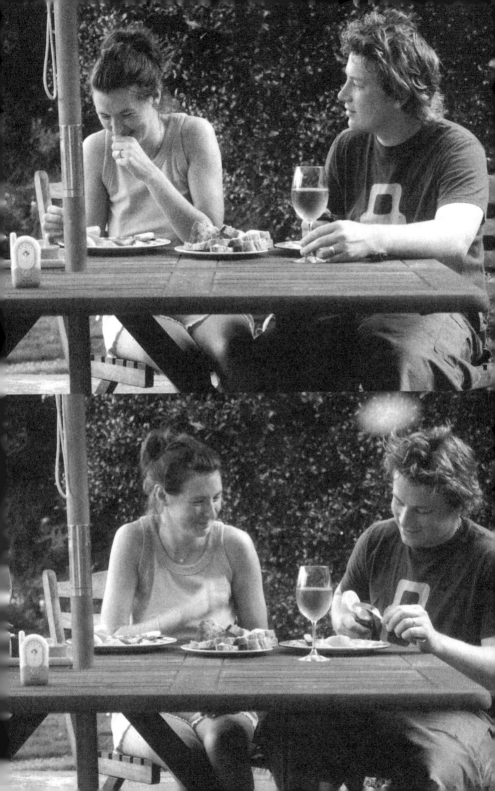

once I loved him for it. With Poppy finally down and fast asleep (and undeniably cute!), the casserole simmering nicely in the Aga and the crumble waiting patiently in the fridge, I had just enough time to decant the mint sauce into a fancy dish and I was done. To be honest, I was pretty damn impressed with myself. Mind you, the only thing that wasn't ready was me. I looked a complete mess. I had flour on my tracksuit bottoms, mint sauce on my T-shirt and let's not even talk about the hair! Too late – he would have to take me as he found me.

When Jamie got home, he was so impressed to be met with his first home-cooked meal in ages, and so happy to see me happy too! Well, I must have impressed him because that night we conceived our second baby and I know for a fact that it wasn't my appearance that won him over, so it must have been my now-infamous lamb casserole . . .
typical chef!

CHAPTER SEVEN

Baby – Three to Six Months

DISCOVERING I WAS PREGGERS WITH DAISY

The last thing on my mind was having another baby . . . well, not just yet anyway. But fate had a hand in that decision!

Poppy was a little over four months old and I finally felt really relaxed as a mum and grateful that life was returning to normal. I had been quite lucky with Poppy, as she had continued to sleep through the night and our routine was really working for us. I had made a few really nice friends from my prenatal classes and our days were spent going for lovely walks or having tea and cakes at each other's houses and generally gossiping and discussing our brood (and, yes, that does include talking in depth about the color and texture of their poo!).

I could even fit into my old jeans, which I am sure is a benchmark for any new mum trying to lose her post-baby weight. Plus, I had finally allowed myself a first night out with Jamie. We went to see a play in the West End and then back to Maxwell's burger bar in Hampstead . . . how romantic! But it meant that we could be close to home (just in case). So, all was well in the Ollie household.

Around about this time I had been planning Poppy's christening. I was loving it, but it felt like it was turning into our wedding all over again with the amount of preparation that was involved. I began to feel really tired and often woke in the morning with that familiar feeling of a turning stomach. I put it down to first-christening nerves, and the tiredness down to all the organizing.

On the morning of the christening I felt really sick but I didn't want to tell anyone and potentially ruin the day, so I carried on as normal (secretly concerned as to why I felt so terrible). It never even entered my mind that I could be pregnant. Before I became pregnant with Poppy, the first classic signs that indicated I might be pregnant had me taking the pregnancy test before you could shout "BABY!" but not this time. Firstly, I was sure that as I was breastfeeding, the likelihood of me conceiving was very slim, and since having sex was always the last thing on my mind after having Poppy, the couple of chances we had managed it just seemed unlikely to me. But most of all I very wrongly assumed, as I had so much trouble conceiving Pops, that next time around it would be the same and I would have to go through the whole ordeal of taking the fertility drugs all over again.

After much thought I decided to take a pregnancy test, seriously believing that I would be wasting my time. It just couldn't be possible. Taking the test this time was a very different experience.

It was a very ordinary morning in the Oliver household. I was about to put Poppy to bed for her morning nap and was going to have a bath myself. I laid her down on her changing mat, about to change her diaper, but decided to take the test then and there. It was only me and Pops in the house, and for once it was really quiet. I nonchalantly peed on the stick, not even bothering to read the instructions this time, and

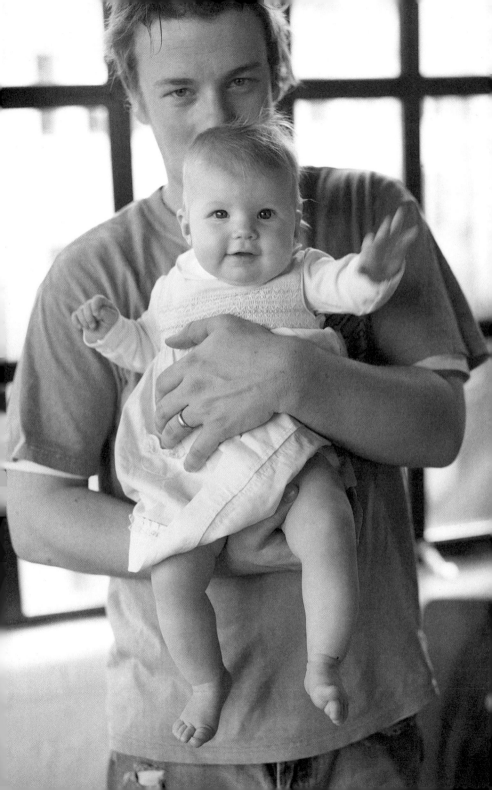

proceeded to change Poppy's diaper, keeping ever such a small eye on the test resting next to me. To my shock, those two blue lines appeared again as if by magic!

So there I was, looking down at my first little baby who was still totally dependent on me in every way. We were still getting used to each other; I was learning so much from her; and I had undoubtedly changed since she had arrived. I really felt I had grown in confidence in every aspect of my life. The moment she entered our lives she was like a mini whirlwind turning everything in our lives upside down – our sleep times, meal times and even our bath times! But she was just perfect, and had enriched our lives tenfold and more. Yet here I was still clutching the positive pregnancy test for another mini whirlwind . . . how would I ever cope?

Telling Jamie I was having another baby happened in much the same way as the first time – he was in a very important meeting and could not be disturbed. Of course, I ignored that and when I finally got through all Jamie could do was laugh. I wasn't sure if this was because he was in a room full of people or whether he was in complete and utter shock, which had sent him into hysteria. I like to think it was the latter! With the initial shock ever so slowly subsiding, I began to feel the familiar surge of excitement that I had when newly pregnant with Poppy.

Suddenly everything had changed. I wanted to step out to get some bread and the simplest thing would have been to put Poppy in her baby sling but then I thought that this could potentially be harmful to the unborn baby, especially as I still had no idea how many weeks along I was. When it came to doing things physically, I had to stop and think about the baby first.

My main worry was that having a second baby so close to the first would mean that neither would receive my full and undivided attention. Poppy had been the center of my world since the day I discovered I was carrying her. I was worried that our close bond would be tarnished, that I would be too wrapped up in baby number two; that Poppy would feel left out, especially near the end of my pregnancy when I was unable to be as active as I would like to have been. I am sure that most women who have had two children close together have all these same feelings. So, this particular section of the book, where I'm writing of Poppy at three to six months, is also the first trimester of my second pregnancy.

BEING PREGNANT SO SOON

It was like starting all over again. It had only been just over four months since I was heaving my big football belly around the house and it was so hard to imagine that I would be doing that all over again in just a few months' time.

I remember how much I used to love taking Poppy out in her baby sling every afternoon, just the two of us. It felt brilliant. We would wander around our village discovering new little cobbled streets and alleyways with coffee shops and interesting houses. It was as if we were discovering things together for the first time. Everything gained a new meaning. (Of course, Poppy was either asleep or dribbling down my T-shirt at the time.) When you start to face your baby outward in the baby carrier (after about eight weeks) it brings a whole new meaning to their world. I know that Poppy loved it.

But all this had to change. I could no longer just throw Pops in the sling and wander around the shops. For starters, it was too tiring carrying a five-month-old baby up the hill to our house and I had no guarantee that it would be safe for my unborn baby to be carrying such a weight around. I felt really disappointed and guilty as I knew Poppy loved the sling.

It's amazing how much you forget the second time around, no matter how long ago you had your first child. The things I can definitely recall are morning sickness with both my babies – I had it up until I was five months pregnant and then intermittently up until they were born. I could just about handle the sickness I had with Poppy, as I could relax in bed until the dreadful feeling had finally subsided, but with Daisy I had no chance for a lie-down because my mornings were normally spent changing a very dirty diaper and vomiting into the toilet – it really was unpleasant and very tiring!

The physical feelings I had had with Poppy were exactly the same as with my second pregnancy, which made me believe that maybe I was having a little girl. However, after my 12-week sonogram, our doctor let slip that there was something going on between the baby's legs which immediately had me thinking we were having a little boy. Of course we were told that this is never a guarantee, especially as it was our first sonogram, but this made no difference to me. I made Jamie do a quick detour on the way home and we stopped off at the nearest baby shop and bought three pale blue sleepsuits and a tiny white-and-blue Grobag (a little sleeping bag for babies)– how wrong were we?

The first three months being pregnant with Daisy were very hard. I constantly felt tired and sick. If these had been the only early problems I would have been very grateful, but they weren't. The first trimester was shockingly different from Poppy's. I thought I had this pregnancy thing in the bag, after all, I had only given birth a few months previously, but I was wrong. Something very unexpected was to happen which threw us all completely off course and turned my otherwise simple and easy pregnancy into a nightmare.

I was about eight weeks pregnant, and, as far as I was concerned, all was well with the baby and me. Jamie had planned a trip to Japan for a week and I was to stay at home with little Poppy. I was dreading him going, as I knew I would miss him terribly. I don't know if it was a new surge of hormones, but I felt incredibly emotional when he had to leave on that Saturday morning.

Everything was as normal as normal could be. I had put Poppy down for her afternoon nap and for the fourth time (due to me drinking large amounts of water!) I went to the bathroom, and realized that I was bleeding. It was such a shock. I didn't think that this ever happened while you were pregnant and therefore assumed that I must be losing the baby. If this has happened to you, you'll know about the instant panic which surged through my body. I literally felt weak at the knees and my face was burning with nervous energy. My first instinct was to call the hospital – although from reading all the countless pregnancy books while I was carrying Poppy, I knew that there was nothing that could be done about early bleeding, especially as I was only eight weeks pregnant. Sitting and riding out the storm was normally all that the doctors and midwives would suggest. I knew that there could be many reasons as to why a woman bleeds during pregnancy: some harmless; others not so. Naturally, I imagined the worst.

As I suspected, the midwife in charge that day merely said that I would have to wait until after the weekend, as it was the Notting Hill Carnival and many staff were off. Crying on the phone, I begged the midwife to just scan me to tell me if my baby's heart was still beating. I know they must receive all sorts of phone calls like this every day, but if it's happening to you, then you need someone on the other end of the phone to at least reassure you. It really is one of the most frightening and scary things I think that can happen while you are pregnant.

The most frustrating and upsetting thing is that there is physically nothing you can do to help the baby, so you feel utterly powerless and have to accept the fact that nature will run its course.

As the hospital was unable to scan me that day, I rushed to the emergency room of my local hospital, leaving Poppy with my sister. It was horrible. I was by myself and in a room full of people all waiting impatiently to be seen. I had desperately tried to get hold of Jamie and left countless messages on his phone, but I feared that he had already taken off and I had missed him. But just as I had given up hope, he called. I was so relieved just to hear his voice. He was about to get ready for take off, but without any hesitation he asked me if I wanted him to come home. All I wanted to do was see him – I needed him with me although it felt selfish to ask him to come all the way back home. But I felt I couldn't go through this alone and I knew he felt the same.

The wait was too long to bear at our local hospital so when Jamie arrived he managed to sort out an emergency appointment at the Portland Hospital. They were brilliant and we were seen straightaway and given a scan.

Reassuringly, we could see that our baby still had a strong heartbeat and that he or she was alive, which was all that mattered to me at that moment.

You may be wondering, after all that, what happened to Jamie and his work trip to Tokyo . . . well, he took a flight out the next day and had a very successful week's work over there opening a new restaurant!

The pregnancy carried on fairly normally after that incident. In fact, it all seemed to go exactly as Poppy's had until about three and a half months. I naturally thought that by now I was out of the danger zone and could happily go through the rest of my pregnancy with no other problems, but I was wrong. The bleeding started again.

It had been a really hot day and I had gone to visit Jamie at the restaurant. I recall feeling really tired, but pushed myself to go out, since Jamie had asked if Poppy and I would join him in a photo shoot for the little Comic Relief book he wrote called *Funky Food*. Pops was still only five months old and I was carrying her everywhere – it was exhausting. After a long shoot I had that horrible familiar feeling that I might be bleeding. I am not sure how I knew but I did. The color

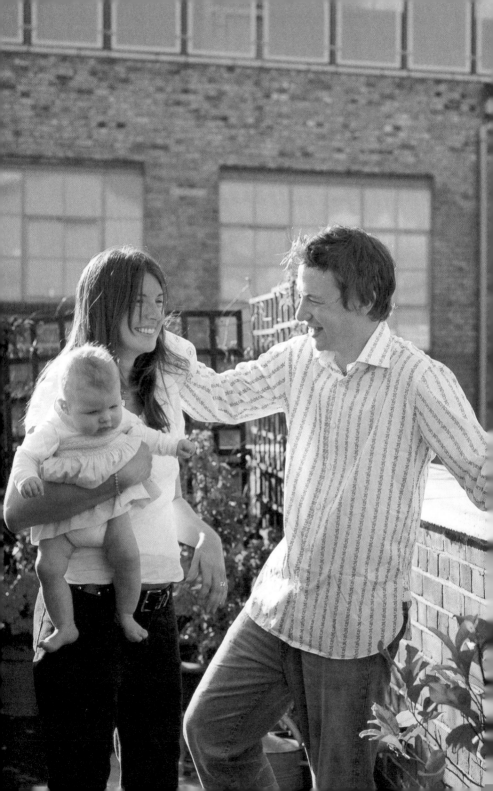

drained from my face and I felt that I had to get to the hospital again, no matter what.

I didn't want to distress Jamie too much, as he had so much work on (and in the back of my mind I hoped that it would be the same procedure as last time) so I told him I was okay to go on my own but that he should leave his phone on and keep it with him just in case.

Luckily my sister Lisa had come along to the shoot with us and drove Poppy and me swiftly to the Portland Hospital, they were able to see me right away. That journey felt like the longest of my life. I kept checking to see if I was still bleeding and each time it seemed to be getting worse and worse. I started to panic, then I started crying and screaming over and over again that I was losing the baby. My sister was amazing. She didn't have a clue where she was going, but she managed to drive as well as reassure me and calm me down, even though she was visibly upset herself. Stuck in traffic, I called Jamie and asked him to come. I needed him – forget work this time! Then I calmly tried to explain to Lisa what she must do with Poppy when I went into the hospital. It's funny what you fuss over when there is an emergency. I was worried about the time as it was past her tea time – the routine was all out of sync! I just wanted to make sure she was taken care of; although I desperately wanted Lisa and Poppy with me, I knew that Poppy should come first.

When we finally arrived I rushed in and garbled out everything to a receptionist. She must have thought I was barmy. I could hardly walk; it was horrendous, embarrassing and so frightening. I stayed in the waiting room on my own, willing Jamie to hurry up, and I remember begging my dad to watch over me and this little baby. Words cannot describe how I was feeling when they finally called me in. I felt weak and was waiting for what I thought would be the news I had been dreading.

The doctor was amazing. She saw my distress and worked quickly. The main thing was seeing the baby on that familiar sonogram machine; hopefully with a little heartbeat.

And there the baby was, moving around, unaware of the distress it was causing its mum. The relief I felt was indescribable. I think I grabbed hold of the doctor's neck and pulled her in for a hug, sobbing on her shoulder. And then Jamie arrived.

While all this had been going on, I had been worried about Poppy, although I knew she was in absolutely safe hands with Lisa. Looking at the time, I imagined that she would be in her pajamas now, having her bottle, and I badly wanted to be with her rather than in hospital. It was probably about then that my fantastic sister walked in with Poppy cuddling into her and I was so happy to see them. As Poppy sucked her thumb and lay on my chest, I was so relieved that she was there. I couldn't be annoyed that she wasn't at home – after all, Lisa had been through hell waiting in the parking lot for me, worrying about me as only a close sister could. I won't forget that. I appreciate and respect my sister in so many ways and love her to bits. I hope that one day Poppy and Daisy will have a similar relationship.

When I first found out that I was pregnant with a second child I wanted to shout it from the rooftops ... after I had got over the initial shock that I was about to do it all over again! But, of course, you never know what's going to happen and so you try and keep it a secret until after your all-clear sonogram at three months. But I can't imagine many mums do – it's just about the most exciting news you can tell someone and holding it back just isn't an option!

Luckily for Jamie and me, this time around we didn't have any journalists or photographers hounding us at our front door demanding that we tell them our baby news. After all, how many journalists would have guessed that three months after giving birth to your first child you would be carrying your second? So, I spent the best part of two months in blissful secrecy with Jamie ... oh, and of course my mum, sisters, best friends, my lovely neighbor, and all of Jamie's family. Oh, and the pharmacist who I bought my pregnancy test kit from ... !

But we knew that we would have to announce it officially at some point. The great thing this time was that we were able to do it the way we wanted to. Jamie had an interview planned with the well-renowned and respected, wonderful journalist Lynda Lee-Potter. She had interviewed Jamie in the past and was the one journalist that he had the ultimate respect for. I remember when she first interviewed him way back at the start of his crazy career. Originally they had been talking about cooking food and the rest, but somehow the conversation had been steered toward family life and me (something which I have always told Jamie to be very guarded about), but after only a short time Lynda and Jamie were chatting away and discussing family like kindred spirits. When Jamie got home that night he told me how he had been interviewed by this wonderful woman who, when discussing my dad and his stroke, had tears in her eyes. Well, we both agreed that you do not get that many sincere people in this world and, I'm sorry to say, certainly not ones that work for newspapers!

So it was inevitable that we would choose to tell Lynda first, officially, of our wonderful news when she interviewed Jamie about his new project – the then unopened restaurant, Fifteen.

We did the interview at our house and Jamie had decided to cook for her as well. We were so nervous. It's not every day that you let members of the press walk freely around your house with a tape recorder! But, as I said, Lynda was different.

In typical Jamie style, he had gone off shopping to Borough Market that Saturday morning and, in even more typical style, was an hour later than he said he was going to be. I had been rushing around tidying the house all morning with Poppy strapped in the baby sling (the only way to stop her crying). It was when I rushed into the village in the blazing hot sun to get flowers that I realized maybe I was going to be struck down with the dreaded morning sickness – yes, it was about that time of year again! As I sat on the pavement with Pops stuck to my chest and a yearning feeling to throw up, I wondered if any minute now there would be a far easier way of telling the world I was pregnant without the use of a journalist!

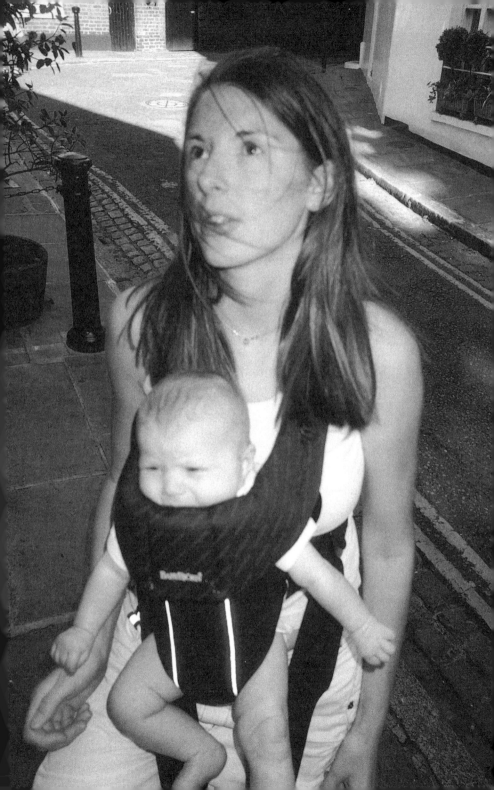

The lunch was a success and telling Lynda was a relief. Judging by my pale complexion and lack of appetite, Lynda, being Lynda, had probably already guessed! Seeing the headline for her article a few weeks later really made it all the more surreal. After all, just three months before – in the same newspaper – Jamie and I had been photographed standing outside the hospital with our first little bundle. And now three were about to become three and a half!

Just recently, and very sadly, Lynda Lee-Potter passed away. For both Jamie and me there will certainly never be a journalist who we will hold in higher regard and respect. She had such integrity and kindness. We will never forget her and I'm so pleased that we both had the pleasure of being interviewed by her and got to call her a friend.

GOING TO BE A MUM AGAIN!

So, with the news out in the open, from that moment on, I was the New Mum Who Was . . . Pregnant! How was I ever going to cope?

This was a wonderful time, as I was really getting used to Poppy and coping with her on my own. I had started to gain confidence, and now that I had become pregnant again, I secretly felt like a true professional. After all, I didn't see many mums wandering around with a three-month-old and a little bump of eight weeks as well! Quite clearly they were sensible enough to use some sort of protection when they re-embarked on their sex lives! Or maybe they have never attempted to cook my ever-so-fertile lamb casserole. Either way, as time went on I was beginning to feel a little less like the supermum and more like the spaced-out, exhausted mum! There was nothing quite like a bout of morning sickness and a morning diaper from Poppy to really put me off ever having kids again.

I remember getting loads of calls and emails from the mums from my prenatal classes who wanted to catch up over coffee and a walk or a shopping spree in town. Feeling as I did, the last thing I thought I could manage was a visit to Oxford Street in the peak of summer. Before any of the mums started asking why I was the most anti-social new mum on the block, I decided to tell my good mate Laura (from my prenatal classes) about my pregnancy. Otherwise I risked losing all my pals for good, and with such a strong network of friends, I definitely didn't want things to dwindle. After all, I was going to be a mum for the second time soon and, since none of my best friends had any babies, I wasn't about to bore them senseless with my tales of baby number two!

So, before Lynda's article was published, it was with a nervous voice that I told Laura the news. After a couple of seconds' silence she whooped with laughter! At first, she thought I was joking; it took a bit of convincing that I was telling her the truth. She was shocked and excited for me, but, as I was later to discover as the news spread fast around the mums, not one of them seemed at all envious . . . I wonder why. . . .

As for Poppy, she was none the wiser. She was obviously getting used to me whipping her off the breast and then seeing me rush into the bathroom to have my timely bout of morning sickness. This was one of the reasons why I wanted to make the transition from breast to bottle, so that her little liquid breakfasts wouldn't be interrupted quite so vigorously!

It was also at about this stage that we decided to try to put Poppy into her own crib in her nursery. I believe the recommended stage to do this with your baby is around the six-month mark, but with Poppy sleeping through most nights we felt that she would really benefit from being in her lovely crib without being constantly interrupted by us coming to bed, switching the lights on and, in most cases, cursing as one of us stubbed a toe on the cradle or tripped over the many toys and accoutrements that Poppy seemed to have gathered on the floor around her sleeping quarters!

So it was with great excitement after her last feed of the day that we carried her up to her little nursery for her first night alone (apart from all the toys and brightly colored mobiles and the giant pink teddy bear which sat proudly in her crib waiting to be loved). I knew she was fond of her room, as we would often hang out in there when the afternoons seemed to last for ages. I didn't think it possible at her age, but Poppy would sometimes look bored, so after taking her out for our usual afternoon stroll and my singing Westlife songs to her on her rug (crikey, no wonder she was bored!) I would head up to her room on the top floor to further entertain her there. Well, what this actually involved was me slumped in her pink spotted armchair desperately trying to keep my eyes open while Poppy lay in her white crib kicking contentedly and cooing animatedly at her "Symphony in Motion" mobile with its sweet classical lullabies.

May I just take some time out here to express my absolute and total gratitude and thanks to whoever invented this

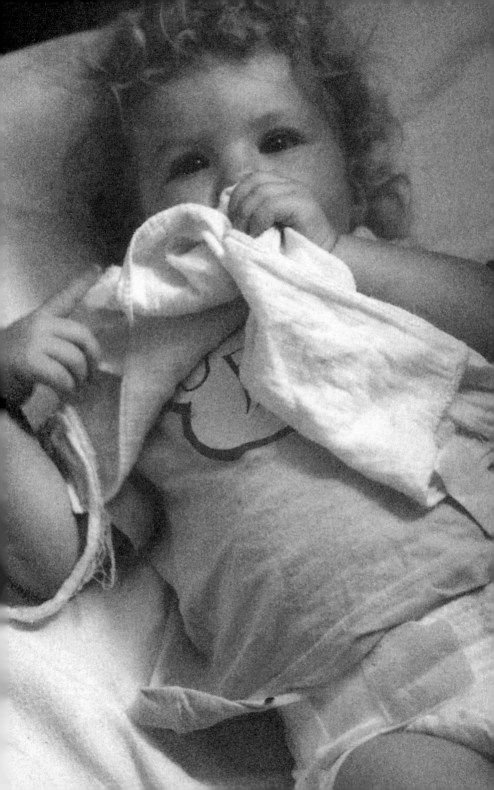

mobile: It really is, was and always will be one of the best things we ever bought both Daisy and Poppy when they were born. If I could, I would dedicate a whole chapter to it, but perhaps that's a little too dramatic. Basically, you can buy beautiful and brightly colored mobiles everywhere but, I believe, nothing quite like this one. As well as having the mobile to hang over the crib, there is a little music box which you attach to the side of the crib and it has three different classical music settings by Mozart, Beethoven and Bach. It comes so highly recommended by me that both my girls still have the music boxes in their rooms (without the mobile attachments now). What really makes us laugh sometimes in the middle of the night is when we hear DJ Dizzy Daisy and DJ Poppy Pops mixing the Mozart decks on a regular basis, choosing their favorite tunes and laying back and relaxing to them; well . . . it makes them happy!

Anyway, so we are on our way to putting Pops snug into her crib. I had lit the room with just her little duck-fairy lights along the wall and her nightlight attached to the monitor. It looked so magical and cozy. My big dilemma was what on earth I should wrap her in once she had graduated from the Moses basket to the crib. At first I had wrapped her in a blanket, all cocooned in white, then after a couple of months when the weather became warmer, I would lay the blanket loosely over her and she would place her arms behind her head so she was free to wriggle during the night. Now we had finally made it to the crib, I was unsure of the bed linen we should be using. On advice from my sister and other mums, the Grobag – like a mini sleeping bag – seemed to be the next stage up in the bedding situation!

So I chose to put Poppy into the smallest Grobag, for babies aged 10 weeks or more, and I placed her in the crib with a simple sheet pulled across the bottom of her feet and tucked it in under the mattress just to keep her in place. Well, she loved it, and on that first night she slept right through and so did we! It was bliss to be able to put the TV on again when we went to bed and, of course, not stub our toes in the dark!

There was the odd night that Poppy would wake up and I would dash up the stairs half asleep, squinting to place myself in the pink spotted chair and breastfeed with my eyes closed. That was the only drawback to feeding Pops in the nursery – it seemed to be more uncomfortable than doing it in the comfort of our warm bed, but hey, you can't have everything!

This whole stage in Poppy's development seemed to just whiz by. I was so consumed with the pregnancy and the breastfeeding and everything else going on that I didn't have time to breathe! It was all so exciting. The things that I definitely do remember were when she reached out for her first object and grasped it in her little fingers. It was her multi-colored triangular wooden toy, and watching the evident determination in her eyes as she tried to focus on the toy and bring it toward her was wonderful. Even though sometimes it might have seemed that my mind and body were in different universes, the joy I received from watching Poppy grow was immense, and it certainly took my mind off some of the distressing times that I had while carrying Daisy.

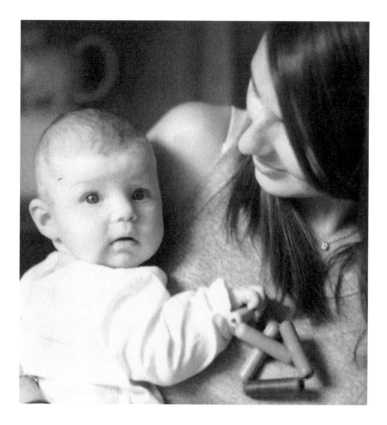

CHAPTER EIGHT

Baby – Six Months to a Year

I absolutely loved this stage of Poppy's life and growth. By the time she was six months old, I really felt relaxed and proud of how I was managing as a mum. With my ever-growing bump and my little plump Poppy – we were a team and I relished the time spent with both of them!

I remember preparing some food for myself one night when Poppy must have been about six months old. She was asleep in the nursery and I'd had some time to read the paper and drink my cappuccino before making myself some dinner. It was still only 7:00 pm and it felt great to have some time to myself, just to do the very mundane and ordinary things that I had taken for granted six months previously! I was speaking to my father-in-law on the phone about this, as I made my roast chicken, and he laughed and reminded me that it wouldn't be long before I had to do it all again. Oh God, I kept forgetting that I was having another BABY!

But for now, I still had to see to all of Poppy's changing needs. The main one at this stage being transitioning her on to solids . . . It was something that I had been dreading for a little while.

POPPY'S FIRST REAL FOOD

When Poppy was almost six months old, as I said above, I felt that I had finally started to settle down into being a mum and that both of us were in quite a good little routine. The breastfeeding was going well and she was sleeping through the night, so I thought that I was doing a pretty good job. But the thing with motherhood is that just as you seem to have everything under control, a new situation arises to throw you completely off balance and you find yourself wading through a whole new set of issues with your baby. I soon began to realize that parenthood is a succession of stages – some exciting, some horrible and some just plain challenging – and that basically it was going to be one long learning curve!

So having settled into our routine, I wasn't really thinking about the next steps to take. It only became apparent that getting her on to solids would be my next hurdle when I joined some of my prenatal class gang on a jaunt to Kenwood House for tea and sympathy! As we sat discussing all the sleepless nights we were having, I noticed that while I was breastfeeding Pops her peers were preparing themselves for a much more grown-up and tasty feast! As the mums pulled out various brightly colored plastic containers, jars and spoons and set about mixing and preparing lunch for their babies I was shocked. When did this stage occur? How come Poppy and I had missed this section of development? (I mean, I know that I wasn't the best at returning emails, and I did have a poor attendance record for these outings, but I started to feel like I had missed a huge chunk of very important bonding somewhere along the line!)

As the mums discussed in great length how much their babies ate, what their favorite meals were, how much rice to add to the dishes and what the best brand of jarred food was to buy, I started to feel extremely left out. I really couldn't contribute to their conversation as I hadn't even thought about introducing solids (well, I had, but it seemed so far off and I was secretly hoping it would never happen!). I felt I had perfected the art of being a mum so well that this might be the proverbial wrench that threw all my hard work off course.

When I returned from the tea party I was crestfallen. I started to panic that I was hindering Pops's development by not having introduced solids to her sooner. I decided to call my health visitor for reassurance and she told me that solids did not actually have to be introduced until your baby was six months old, and that if Pops was sleeping through the night she was obviously getting enough food and nutrients from my breast milk, so I was not to stress about it at all.

But right now I needed a bit of direction – I was too tired to think for myself and all I wanted was to be given a date to work toward. But, of course, that was not possible. Again, it was down to "mother's instinct" – oh God, not that old chestnut again! In fact it was kind of a gradual thing for me and with a little of that precious instinct I decided to move to the next step and start weaning Pops.

If you are anything like me (a worrier, a slight dramatist and a panicker) you will understand these next couple of paragraphs!

Upon extensive reading of my countless books, I discovered that in order to start the weaning process properly and more easily you had to own a sterilizer. Having solely breastfed Poppy, I didn't have a clue how to use one. I had initially bought an electric one in my pre-baby shopping spree just in case I was unable to breastfeed and would be using bottles instead. I was so nervous about this sterilizing and when I think back to how I was feeling it makes me laugh – how ridiculous, it was hardly rocket science!

I decided to test the sterilizer out one night so I put all the bottles, nipples, weaning spoons, plastic plates, rattles, and basically anything that moved, into the machine. Following the instructions carefully, I watched the thing like a boiling kettle. After eight minutes I checked that the yellow light had gone off (about 100 times) then set about taking everything out and setting it up as if it was real. Using the little tweezers that come with the sterilizer, so that you DON'T TOUCH any of the baby equipment, was never going to be easy, as I was so nervous. A nipple sprang out of the pincers and flew across the room – oh SHIT! Did this mean that I had to go through the whole tiresome process again? Also, once I had everything out, did this mean that the items were no longer sterile for Poppy to use in the morning? This was all so confusing and I was stressing out all on my own (Jamie, on the other hand, found all of this a piece of cake . . . naturally!). However, I shouldn't have worried because once the bottles had their lids on they would stay sterile until I came to use them the following day – easy as that. And after a little more practice and less worrying, I soon came to realize that if I did drop something on the floor it could be rinsed with boiling water from kettle to sterilize it quickly instead of having to go through the whole rigmarole of the sterilizer again.

After extensive practice sessions I had the whole sterilizing process sorted out. So, using Annabel Karmel's *New Complete Baby and Toddler Meal Planner,* I set about giving Poppy her first taste of real food, or rice as it's more commonly known in the baby world! This simply involved mixing two teaspoons of baby rice with about four teaspoons of baby milk formula or expressed breast milk and mixing it into a soft paste. I used to use a plastic lid from one of the bottles as a little bowl – it was the perfect size and I could easily chuck it into the sterilizer afterward. I found it was handy to prepare the little bottle of formula milk first, say the night before, and pop it in the fridge so all I had to do then was warm it up and mix it with the rice. I think the key, especially with these initial stages, is to be extremely organized, if you can. The last thing you need is a screaming hungry baby while you're running around trying to will the sterilizer to HURRY UP – they just don't understand!

With all this build-up, it was weird to be giving Poppy just two tiny teaspoons of what looked like wallpaper paste. And half of it fell out of her mouth and half landed on me! She would roll it around her mouth and spit it back out again and so the lengthy process of her pushing it out of her mouth, and me spooning it back in, could take up to 15 minutes just for two mouthfuls. It was a very messy process!

Now all this seemed straightforward, but what confused me was the concept of weaning. When should I actually stop giving Poppy my breast milk and just give her solids and at what times of the day should I feed her? I had so many unanswered questions.

For the first week I started off by simply giving her one meal of rice at about 10:45 am followed by her usual amount of breast milk afterward, before her afternoon nap at midday. She seemed to be fine with that, so on the second week of following the simple routine laid out in Annabel Karmel's book, I upped her rice feeding to twice a day, by including one at around 4:00 pm. This came in between her milk feed at 2:30 pm and her last milk feed of the day at 6:00 pm.

So, after two weeks, and with the first stage successfully out of the way, I soon realized that there was a harder one just around the corner. It was time for the real McCoy – I was going to have to start making actual food! I had really gotten into mixing up the baby rice and milk and was enjoying the routine and here we were – off again to do something different!

After studying my books extensively, and chatting to various mums, I realized that the most popular choice for a baby's first solid meal was pureed carrot. I thought it was probably best to start off with a savory one first in case she developed a sweet tooth like her mum – now that really wouldn't be good!

Okay, fantastic, I knew roughly how to cook carrots! The night before Poppy's big feast, I played around in the kitchen preparing the carrots. I know this all must sound silly – I am sure as you're reading this you're thinking "how hard can cooking some carrots be? What a fuss!" In fact, as I'm writing this I'm thinking the same thing, but at the time it was a real landmark for me as a mum.

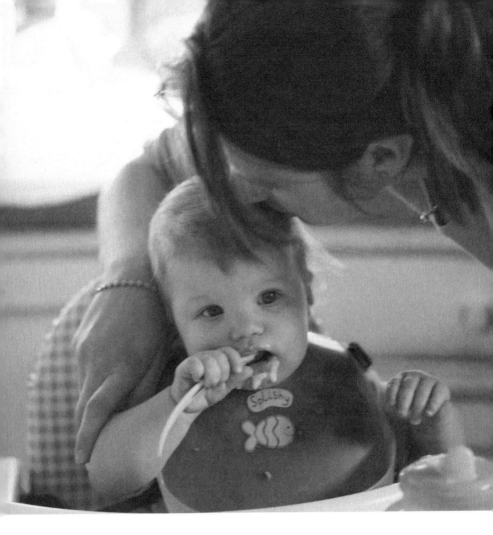

I wasn't sure if I had to sterilize all my cooking utensils, including the saucepan – how does one fit that into the sterilizer? So, after scorching myself while pouring boiling water over all the utensils I planned to use, I felt ready to boil up some carrots! After mashing them into a very smooth puree, I poured them into my waiting ice-cube tray . . . brilliant! It was all going according to the book (although it failed to mention that the whole process would take an hour or so – or maybe that was just me). Then I gleefully placed my orange-colored trays into the freezer and spent the next five hours checking on them as if they were the crown jewels!

I was excited about Jamie coming home that night as I knew that he would be proud of me . . . this is all sounding a bit ridiculous now, after all I wasn't a culinary dunce in the kitchen. Far from it; judging by my "carrots à la freezer" I was a culinary genius! As I proudly showed off my frozen cubes, I knew that Jamie would have to have a little input into my finished dish. It wasn't long before he was suggesting that I chop up a few fresh herbs like basil or mint to mix in with the carrot (chefs just can't help themselves).

The excitement as I heated up Poppy's carrot cube was infectious. Both Jamie and I were very well prepared – me with an apron covering me from head to toe (I knew I was in for a messy ride) and Jamie with his video camera, Polaroid camera and various other long-lensed cameras around his neck (I knew we had all angles covered!).

I decided that it would be best to prop Poppy up in her baby bouncer in front of me. Well, she loved it! No sooner had I given her one mouthful than her little mouth opened again like a baby bird wanting more. I was so happy that she liked the food!

FOOD ON THE MOVE

At around this time we had booked a short break away for a few days in a hotel near Bath – just the three of us. I wondered if I should just ditch the food thing until we returned, as I wasn't sure I could face taking along all the food equipment paraphernalia with us, but with encouragement from Jamie I decided that, as we had taken this new step and she seemed so enthusiastic about it, we should carry on. But how would I keep all my carrot cubes fresh? It would mean that I was going to have to buy jarred baby food, which to me was disappointing. I had wanted to start her off on completely fresh food (that way I knew exactly how it had been prepared, what was in it, and so on). But it was too complicated, so jars it was.

Looking at the array of jars available to buy, I was confused. They all looked basically the same – all the carrot varieties were orange with a very smooth consistency – so how was I to tell which one would be best? I eventually decided to go with the Baby Organix brand – mmmm, delicious!

We were into Day 2 of Week 3 – renamed "carrot week" as she had moved on from the baby rice! Feeding Poppy in our hotel was a whole new ball game. If you are a mum or dad already, you will understand how difficult it is to go away with a young baby and all the stuff that you have to take with you – you can't help it! You don't want to be left outside your comfort zone, and that can apply to anything from a short walk to the shops, to a holiday abroad. When we got out of our car at the hotel, it was obvious that our days of two small weekend bags were over! Now we had three weekend bags; one baby-bouncer chair; a play gym; three baby blankets; sheets and Grobags; an impressive array of rattles, cuddly toys and other wooden accoutrements, which I swore were her favorites, and we couldn't leave home without them. With hindsight, I don't think that she gave a damn about any of them – they were my safety blankets more than anything. Not forgetting the all-important burping cloths for cleaning up various baby spills and also for Poppy to snuggle up to. (Her new thing was to suck her thumb while holding a cloth next to her nose.) So, we were carrying all that with us, not to mention the mini sterilizer, spoons, sippy cups, baby rice, jars and dishes. I won't even go into the number of diapers and wipes we took, but everything managed to fit into our small hotel room. Thank goodness they provided a travel crib or we were going to have to resort to buying the minivan five years too early – I don't think Jamie was quite ready for that life-changing experience just yet!

Anyway, we made it into our hotel room and it was time once again to feed Poppy. In a new environment with limited supplies, I decided to take the advice of my big sis and stick to feeding Poppy one thing for about four days to see if she liked it and also, more importantly, to see if anything gave her an unfavourable reaction. That way we would know exactly which food it was and could eliminate it for a while and reinstate it a little further down the track when her taste buds had changed. So, carrots it still was, in the morning, and baby rice in the afternoon.

Now there was one thing which did change at this stage and that was the color of Poppy's poo. As you might expect, it no longer resembled smooth mustard but became more like a proper poo! I know that this all sounds so unpleasant but I have to admit that in my naivete as a first-time mum, I did wonder how solid food was going to affect her bowel movements. I was quite excited to see this new change occur – it was another mini milestone in Poppy's life, so to me it was completely fascinating! However, I can categorically say that I am no longer fascinated by Poppy's (or Daisy's) poo and cannot change a diaper or pair of panties fast enough!

So that was it. Poppy was now officially a baby on solids, although a little later than her little friends. I was glad that we were past the first hurdle. Along the way there were hundreds of things that I didn't understand or have a clue how to do. Simple things like quantities of puree and how many cubes should I defrost the night before? In the end, I would freeze a huge batch in one go and would usually do two ice-cube trays of pureed carrots, two of zucchini-and-spinach puree and then, for a change, I would puree some sweet apples and pears in another tray. Then each night I would take out two cubes and defrost them in the fridge in a little plastic container. That would suffice for her lunch (you can always add some baby rice with a little formula or breast milk if you want to bulk it out, especially if your little one seems to be a hungrier baby).

Another thing I wasn't sure about was when to start introducing the second ice cube "meal" of the day, so I decided to ditch the afternoon rice feed about three or four weeks after I had introduced her first meal and set about offering her two sweet cubes (apple and pear, or apricot and raspberry) or just simple mashed banana, papaya or mango. She loved all of these fruits and ate them with gusto. I sometimes added baby rice to bulk them out and make her feel fuller. Poppy loves her fruit now and out of pure habit I still give her some after her tea as her dessert – she adores it. I attribute this to her early introduction to such a variety of it.

The next question was, when do I introduce a second course at mealtimes? Well, I think after about six or seven weeks of Poppy being on solids twice a day, I started to introduce desserts to her meal times so at lunch she would have maybe two or three cubes of vegetables followed by a little baby yogurt, then at dinnertime she would have another serving of vegetables and maybe a little baby pasta, with two fruit cubes for dessert. It was a gradual process with her leading the way – it's definitely worth following your baby's lead as to how much they want to eat. My girls were never particularly hungry babies and, as they both slept through the night quite early on, it was hard for me to know when they wanted to up their food or milk intake. For example, during most breastfeeds, both Poppy and Daisy would feed from just one breast for only about three or four minutes per session. There was the odd time when they would feed for up to an hour, but usually it was little and often. So I expected the same when it came to solids. They ate what I gave them but never really screamed for more (which was handy!).

The next thing to tick off on the list of solids was adding breakfast to the agenda. This came a few more weeks down the line, and soon I found myself eating my breakfast at 7:00 am along with Pops, spooning one mouthful of baby cereal with mashed banana into her mouth and one spoonful of whatever I could find into mine. Everything was changing and I think I was handling it all okay so far!

BREAST TO BOTTLE

The next big issue, which was all part of the weaning process, was moving Poppy from the breast to the bottle. I had wanted to exclusively breastfeed her until she was about six or seven months old, but as nature had stepped in and I was growing another baby inside me, I was worried that the breastfeeding might affect the pregnancy. I've since found out that it would have been fine to have carried on, as long as I had increased my fluid intake. I was also extremely tired in the early stages of my second pregnancy and this was partly due to my breastfeeding. As Poppy was now six months old and doing really well with her solids, I knew that I should start to ease her off the usual four milk feeds a day, and up the amount of solid food that she was having. It just seemed so complicated though – how was I to know when to lessen the milk and by how much? As far as I was concerned, Pops loved both her milk and her food. Again, it was a matter of gradual change so that neither of us was particularly aware that anything had chang so first of all I needed to get Poppy off the boob and on to the bottle. . . .

One afternoon I decided to take the plunge and sterilize a nipple and a bottle and fill it with the baby formula. I had tried this process a long time before, when Poppy was about two months old and Jamie had wanted to feed her himself – I'd sterilized a bottle and expressed some breast milk. I

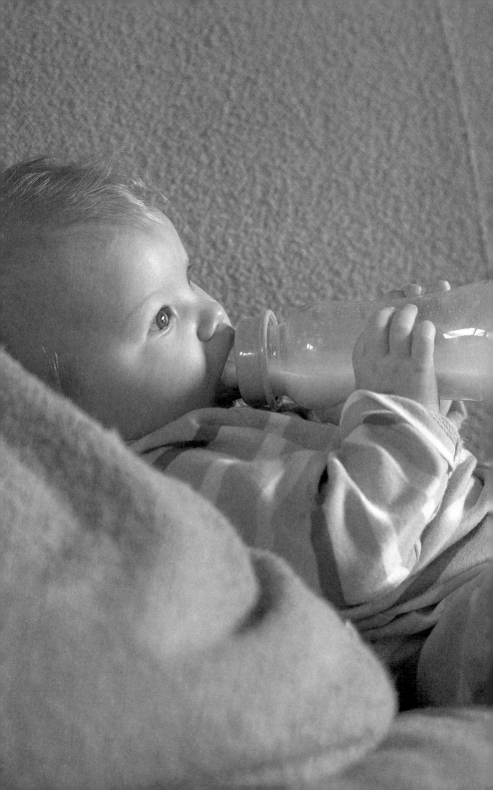

found it such a hassle, though, as I never knew at what time of the day I had the most milk and I didn't want to use up my supplies on a little bottle which I had no guarantee that she would take anyway. I did find this stage to be one of the most complicated points of being a mum yet!

Well, I can only tell you that I did it in my own way. And what seemed like a terribly complicated step did turn out to be fairly painless for both of us. Poppy was already successfully drinking cooled boiled water from a little sippy cup with her meals, but had not quite graduated to the bottle. So the first job was to choose what type of bottle to use. There were two main brands on the market that I was interested in – Avent and Nuk. The Avent range is widely available and the nipple are generally wider and fatter than other brands and very closely resemble a mum's nipple. The Nuk bottles and nipples were far more slender and I found that Poppy took to them more quickly. Well, I say quickly but it took me about six weeks to finally get her exclusively on to the bottle – and it was quite hard work.

As part of my daily routine, I sterilized my bottles and made up some formula for her last feed of the day. It was 7 oz. and I only knew how much to do by looking at the back of the baby formula packet (Hipp Organic if you are interested). It had a very helpful chart outlining how many ounces to give your baby at each feed according to their age – it was a godsend, as I didn't have a clue how much breast milk Poppy was getting – it certainly didn't feel like 7 oz.! Every night I would settle her down after her bath, all snuggled up in her Grobag, to have her bottle, and each time she rejected it. It was so disappointing. Eventually the guilt would set in and I would give in to her gut-wrenching cries for my breast. As she guzzled on my boob, contented at last, I felt lost. Was she ever going to give me up? Would I be breastfeeding Poppy in the morning before she set off for school? Help! – why wasn't it working? Bottle after bottle would be thrown away. I even tried to change the times for her to have the bottle – either first thing in the morning or just before lunch – thinking that perhaps she was just too tired after her bath and the last thing she wanted was a plastic nipple shoved down her throat. But each time she rejected it and wouldn't give in.

It was suggested to us that Jamie, or someone else close, should try and feed her, because she could smell my milk, and therefore would never want the bottle. This was harder than it sounds, as Jamie was always working late and sometimes on the weekends. No, I was determined to do this myself. It had now become my mission. I decided to bind myself up in one of Jamie's sweatshirts to try and mask the smell of my milk, and one day, after six weeks of trying, she took the bottle and started drinking. She didn't stop till she had finished the whole thing and I didn't move for ages, convinced that if I breathed or even moved my feet I would distract her and she would remember there was more delicious milk elsewhere. I don't know why that night was different to any other – maybe I was more relaxed at this point and not expecting it. I was elated that the breakthrough had finally happened. I knew that this was going to free me up somewhat and change my life again!

I still carried on breastfeeding Pops during the day and was always relieved when the time came to give her the bottle at night. It felt so weird and wonderful to be able to relax while she contentedly drank her milk. I would watch TV or read a magazine, happy that I no longer had to hunch over her like Quasimodo. I could also now see exactly how much milk she was having. At the beginning I would top her up with my heavier boob. But after a while she no longer required my extra breast milk and seemed wholly satisfied with her formula. The battle with the bottle was won!

The weaning process was nearly over – all I had to do now was gauge how much Poppy was eating every day and then lessen her milk once she was on three meals a day. Her milk intake had gone down to 6 oz. in the morning and 7 oz. before bedtime. She still had an additional bottle of about 4 oz. at mid-morning before her lunch, then another of about 3 or 4 oz. at around 2:30 pm after her afternoon nap. But these soon became pointless, as very often she would suck on the nipple for a minute then roll the bottle across the floor. Every night I would have to search under the sofa for cold bottles of formula! It looked like all the food and extra water I had given her had completed the weaning process successfully but it had all been quite a task.

LUMPY FOOD

After your baby has been on solids for a while, you will have to start thinking about lumpiness and when should you move them up a notch to deal with more solid solids. With Poppy I was very cautious about moving her quickly on to lumpier foods because I was really concerned that she might choke. Being unable to perform the Heimlich maneuver, it frightened me to death, but at the same time I didn't want her to get used to only eating smooth purees as I'd have another problem on my hands later on! Luckily I met a wonderful girl named Becci who is a professional nanny. She came to work for me one morning a week so I could get some rest, but naturally I never rested (if it wasn't the washing that I was grappling with, I would find myself chatting to Becci while she looked after Pops). Becci taught me a lot about the feeding issues and gave me the confidence I needed to move forward and try new things with Poppy.

With Becci there, I was lucky enough to have a little time on my hands to experiment and learn more about the food part of a baby's development. Being married to a chef, it was only natural that I should be interested in the subject. I decided quite early on that I wanted to try and feed Poppy with home-cooked and, where possible, organic food. It was always going to be one of the most important issues to us as parents. So, every week I would set about doing a big cook-off, as I called it, for Poppy and then I'd freeze all the food into little ice-cube trays in the freezer. If Jamie was around when I was doing this, he'd "interfere" a little bit at the

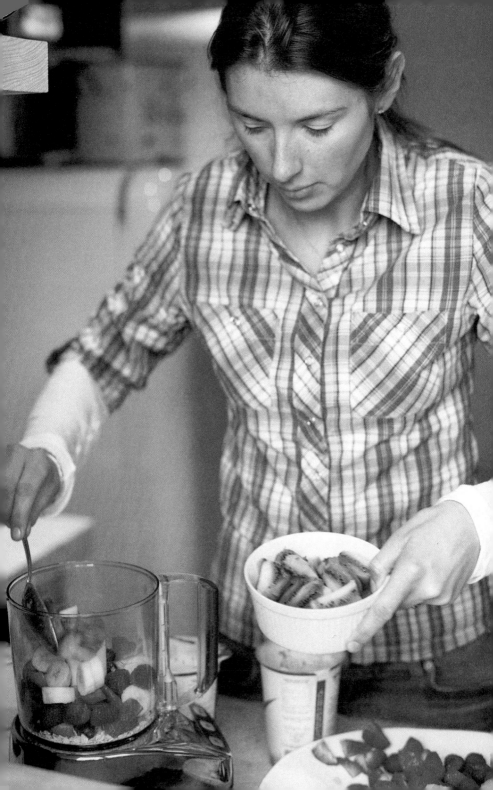

beginning, suggesting different combinations of veg, for instance, but nothing more than that. I kept things basic for the first few months though.

As I said earlier in this chapter, I set about pureeing carrot at first, but then I moved on to all sorts of different fruits and vegetables. Poppy would eat butternut squash, zucchini and leeks, then apples, pears, apricots and peaches. These foods were obviously quite easy to prepare as they pureed well and kept for up to three months in the freezer. As time went on, I got a bit cocky and started combining things like peas, zucchini and fresh mint. Both my girls LOVED this combination. I then introduced strawberries and raspberries for their bright colors and lovely texture – Pops loved them.

Sometimes I would combine, say, two pureed chicken cubes with two vegetable ones of any sort and defrost them in separate tubs. Then, when needed, I could heat them up and have a really quick, easy and nutritious meal ready in seconds. The same applied to the sweet snacks – three little cubes of fruit puree in a container defrosted the same way.

With encouragement from Becci, I started to make the food a little lumpier. Poppy was about eight months by now and I did find it a lot easier. There was no need to whizz anything up in the food processor now – I could simply mash it all with a fork. I was very proud of my cooking for Poppy and had really started to enjoy it as well – something I NEVER thought would happen!

As time went on, and I became more tired with my second pregnancy, my enthusiastic cook-offs became rarer and rarer. Instead, as I invariably ate on my own at night, I would make

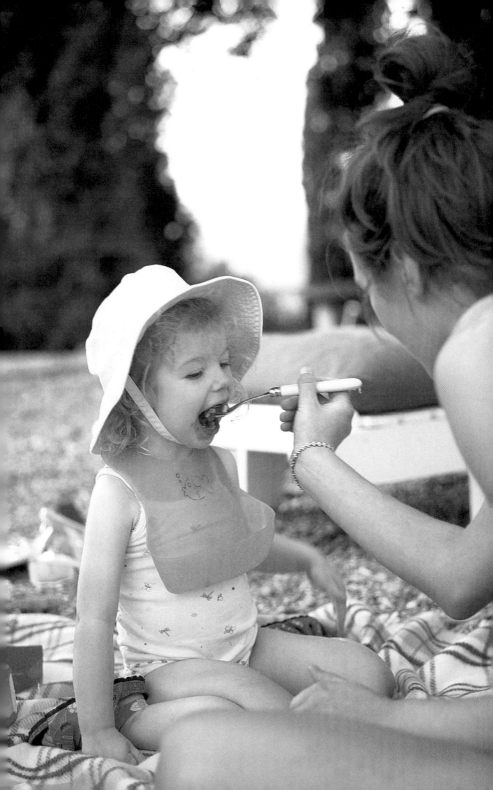

my dinner and before seasoning it with any salt I would put some on a plate for Poppy and reheat it for her the next day. This didn't happen every night, but usually on the occasions that I was having fresh minestrone, or fish and vegetables, or chicken casserole (all of which taste better the next day anyway), and she loved them too! I soon became pretty good at cooking for her and, on Jamie's insistence, became more experimental as well. I think that Poppy probably had more flavors and transatlantic ingredients in her food in one year than I have had in my whole life! Ironically, though, she went through a fussy stage when she got to about a year old, where she would prefer to eat, for example, a plain bit of fish with some peas, rather than having any nice sauce with it. This lasted on and off for a while, and even now she has opinions on what she likes and dislikes.

AND SO IT WAS TIME TO LABOR AGAIN ...

When Poppy was a year old, I was due to have my second child. It was early April, and I was seven days overdue. Again, I thought that this one would be early so I was very well prepared! I had had my labor bag packed for more than two months – it was sitting in the spare room, which was slowly being transformed into Poppy's new bedroom. The new baby was going to move into Poppy's old room.

I had been bleeding lightly for about five days, but was less worried about it with this baby. I felt so much more confident this time around and felt more relaxed about certain things. But nonetheless I was really ready to pop with the pressure that was mounting from the constant stream of paparazzi who would "hide" behind the line of sycamores opposite our house with their zoom lenses poking out. I think that they expected me to dramatically give birth then and there on the pavement every time I walked out of my front door. Rather unfortunately for them, the only pictures they will have managed to get are of me putting out the garbage bags, or struggling to put Poppy into her stroller, or walking down the road carrying a shopping bag . . .

STRETCH AND SWEEP

I didn't really want to be induced, as I was hoping that labor would start naturally, so it was suggested by my wonderful obstetrician (the same man who delivered Poppy) that before we resort to an inducement he should carry out a procedure called a "stretch and sweep." Now, I know that this sounds weird. In fact, my friend Lindsey, who was pregnant at the same time as me, thought that it was an aerobic exercise that you did with your doctor to help bring on the birth! If you're still wondering what on earth it means, have a look at the glossary entry on page 283, but to give you a brief idea it's an internal examination where the doctor stretches your uterus to try and start labor! I know a lot of women decline to have this done but I was happy to try anything to bring the labor on and to avoid any unnatural intervention. The doctor was convinced that I would go into labor naturally, so he allowed me to go over my due date by 10 days before thinking about inducing me.

After my usual blood pressure and other regular checks

it was time for the sweep. I had conjured up all sorts of ridiculous images about this while trying to sleep the night before and I was quite nervous. I had a fear of the unknown, but I can honestly say that it was absolutely fine. The best way to describe it was like having a Pap smear which was just a little more thorough than usual!

I was shocked to find out that I was actually about 3 cm dilated already and I hadn't even known it. And to think that when I'd been in labor with Pops, at 3 cm I was climbing the walls in pain and begging for an epidural. The only walls I had been climbing so far with this labor were at Brent Cross Shopping Centre where I'd been scanning the rails for last-minute goodies! So, with my sweep swept, it was now just a question of waiting to see if it had worked.

As a little treat, Jamie decided to take me shopping. I was excited at the prospect of a) spending time with him on a clandestine shopping trip when he should have been at work, and b) a trip to our favorite antique shop in Primrose Hill. However, after the morning's events I felt less enthusiastic than I would normally have been, and more tired than ever. I was also, dare I admit it, feeling a slight nagging pain down below – a little bit like contractions, but I couldn't be sure. This time around I was determined to hold on for longer before going to the hospital as I wanted to labor in the comfort of our own home, so I kept quiet. As we wandered around Primrose Hill (or should I say "waddled"), I began to realize that perhaps I WAS actually in labor. Jamie was called away on urgent business and, for once, I was relieved that we had to end a shopping trip prematurely.

When I got home I called the doctor and explained to him what I was experiencing. He thought that it might be because of the sweep and suggested that I carry on my day as normal. But I knew something was different. I sat down to watch *This Morning* (is there a repetitive theme here?) and my sister Lisa made me a delicious lunch of tomato pasta. She warned me that there was heaps of garlic in it but I was too hungry to care, so I wolfed it down (something that I later came to regret). By 2:30 pm I knew that I was in labor. The pains I was having were just too regular and similar to be anything else. I called Jamie and told him, but he was reluctant to leave work and tried to convince me that it was a false alarm. He was about to go into a meeting in Hammersmith with the second round of students for his restaurant Fifteen. We were laughing on the phone, as he was sure that we were in for the long haul and that our second baby would take two days, just like Poppy, but after much deliberation he decided to cancel the meeting and come home.

When he arrived I was having my usual pre-labor bath! This time though, I had a little partner in the form of Poppy. Lisa was filming me in the bath, trying to capture the birthing experience from start to finish (something that I hadn't done with Poppy and since regretted). She was asking me all these annoying questions, as sisters do, and making me laugh, which was becoming increasingly difficult as the contractions were picking up speed and it was getting uncomfortable. It's hilarious to watch it now – the pain etched on my face as I tried to shave my legs with an over-excited 13-month-old laying on my tummy is quite a picture, and the size of my boobs and belly . . . ! I am surprised that

Poppy even fit into the bath with me. My obstetrician, Dr. McCarthy, called me at this point to tell me that as this was my second baby I should really be in the hospital as there was a likelihood that it would arrive much faster than the first. With that said, I was out of the bath and racing downstairs to tell Jamie. Undeterred by my dramatic naked entrance and declaration that we were off to the hospital, Jamie carried on watching a film and suggested that I lay down next to him and relax whilst he massaged my feet . . . was he joking? There was no time. I called John, a friend of ours, to ask if he would pick us up and suddenly it was action stations for everyone. Apart from Jamie – he kept insisting that we all settle down and finish the film, before calmly making our way to the hospital. Ignoring him, I lugged my labor bag down from the third floor, cursing him all the way. He finally got the message when he saw me clinging on to the fireplace and breathing like a long-distance runner.

On the way to the hospital, I called my eldest sister, Nat, for last-minute advice on having a second baby. In between the contractions I asked her how painful it might get – I had no idea how much I had dilated, but I thought that I probably hadn't quite reached my full pain threshold just yet anyway! Jamie decided that now was a good time to start the "daddycam" and film a blow-by-blow account of his version of becoming a father for the second time. This included filming the paparazzi who had decided that following a woman in labor might just give them the money shot they had been waiting nine months for! It was like a car chase scene from a movie. Not only was John trying to negotiate the busy route to the hospital with me screaming out directions, but under Jamie's instruction he was also trying to dodge the photographers by taking a different route than mine. You can only imagine the pandemonium in that car.

It was nearing four o'clock when we finally reached the hospital. We saw about 16 paparazzi guys jump out of their cars to get in front of us and do the rest on foot . . . the BASTARDS. Crouching in my seat I continued having full-on contractions, hoping that no one could see. Jamie, meanwhile, had instructed John to carry on driving to try and lose them . . . for goodness sake – lose them where? I had to go into the hospital eventually. Was he expecting me to give birth in the car? (I am sure John was hoping otherwise.)

When I finally got out of the car, I just lost it in mid-contraction. I flew at the photographers and yelled something very rude. I felt so cool, like Liam Gallagher. These two separate words were all it took for them to stop in their tracks and actually look slightly guilty as I limped into the hospital. I felt totally jubilant, until I heard Jamie. He had seen me upset and had taken action to protect me a little too late as I was almost halfway to the ward. He shouted out, "Come here, you little p***k, before I punch you, come here." Oh God, here we go, I thought. As I glanced behind me, I was just in time to see Jamie swinging my handbag over his shoulder, brandishing it like a baton, the hospital doors automatically opening and closing behind him. He then did a very impressive *Karate Kid*-style high kick which Sporty Spice would have been proud of! It was hilarious and really put a smile back on my face; I needed this little light relief to get me through. We found out afterward that the camera had been shoved back into my handbag with the lens cap on but the sound still recording, so we have all this for posterity!

With all this drama it was no surprise that when I finally lay down on my hospital bed and had the monitor strapped to my tummy my contractions began to waver. They no longer felt as painful as before. I was also 4 cm dilated – I didn't know whether to laugh or cry!

As a precaution, it was decided that I would be taken to the delivery room just in case there was a sudden change. There I was met by Dr. McCarthy who suddenly made me feel totally at ease and very calm. He went through the usual procedures with me and said, judging by looking at me, that we still might have some time before the baby arrived.

Once Jamie and I were left alone and I had changed into my T-shirt and funky slippers (which my lovely mum-in-law had bought me for this purpose) we settled in to watch a bit of TV, but all too soon the contractions started up again. As soon as Dr. McCarthy actually watched me having a contraction he knew that the birth was imminent, but not even we imagined that it would be as quick as it was. After 15 minutes of walking up and down the hallway, under the instruction of the midwife (I personally didn't want to do this as I could hear the howls and wails from the other rooms coming at me from all directions), I decided I would much rather be in my bed watching a bit of early evening TV, privately wailing through my own contractions.

I was hoping to use a birthing pool at some point as I had heard that being in water can really help you to cope with the pain, so I asked a midwife if she could fill a pool for me to relax in. As I hobbled to the bathroom with Jamie in tow, suddenly something changed. I felt like I needed to go to the bathroom, RIGHT NOW! How horrifying. I wasn't sure if it was that or the baby's head but I felt this incredible pressure to push – something which I didn't experience with Poppy's birth because of the epidural. Bearing in mind that we had only been at the hospital for an hour, I started to go into shock. This couldn't be right. I thought that I must get back to my room so I could get my epidural. It was the most incredible sensation. As I watched the midwife clean the bath (that's what the "pool" was), my normal polite self suddenly turned into an animal. Forget the bath! I had to lie down before this baby fell out! I practically ran from the bathroom into the hallway, clutching my crotch for dear life and running, as Jamie described it, like John Wayne in a western!

I threw myself on to the bed, panicking as I tried to get my underwear off. The last thing I wanted now was to hinder my baby on the way out. My water was then broken by the midwife, as I was at 10 cm and it was still intact. I couldn't believe that I had progressed from 4 to 10 cm in an hour! It was all happening so quickly. I began to feel delirious – this wasn't helped by the gas and air, which I hadn't wanted, but I was now sucking on it like it was a strawberry daiquiri! I then began to spout nonsense to Jamie and Dr. McCarthy. They must have thought I was mad. Even as I was pushing I was screaming out that I didn't want a caesarean. I was so disoriented that I didn't even flinch when I realized that all that pushing had made me – horror of horrors – do a POO!

This had been one of my nightmare scenarios if ever there was one, but let me tell you that when you're going through this experience it really is the last thing on your mind!

What I found amazing was being able to actually feel everything that was happening to my body. At one point the midwife explained that I might be entering what they call in the business the "ring of fire" ... need I say more? It meant that the baby's head was crowning – no wonder I was yelping like a puppy! In between the contractions, my whole body would relax and I was even able to have light conversation, although I doubt that what I was saying made much sense. While Jamie mopped my brow, waved a fan over my face and gave me sips of water I, in return, bit his hand, wrung his wrists and pulled his hair so hard that I managed to drag his whole body under the bed. It really was the only way to cope with the pain! Little did I know that all this was being recorded for Jamie's mini epic and could be used against me at any time in a future argument! During these abusive moments, Jamie looks right at the camera capturing everything as if it were a real cinematic moment.

After only 35 minutes of actual pushing, our beautiful little Daisy Boo was born. She was put straight on to my chest and, unlike Poppy, she cried immediately. With her little mop of dark hair I fell in love with her at once!

X

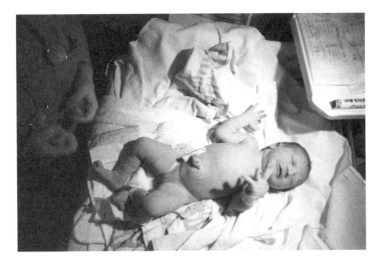

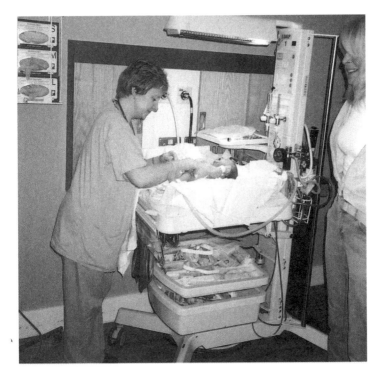

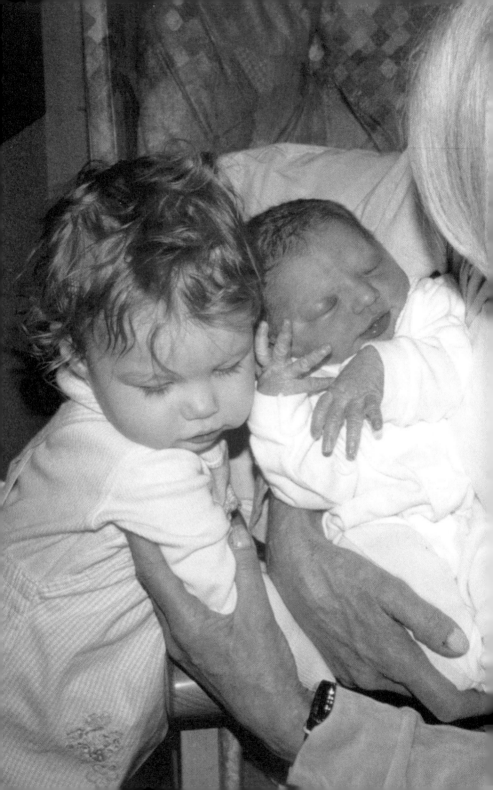

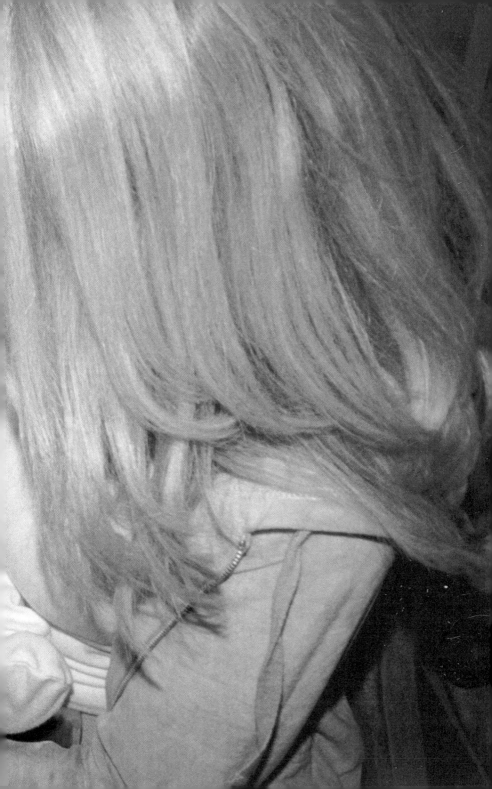

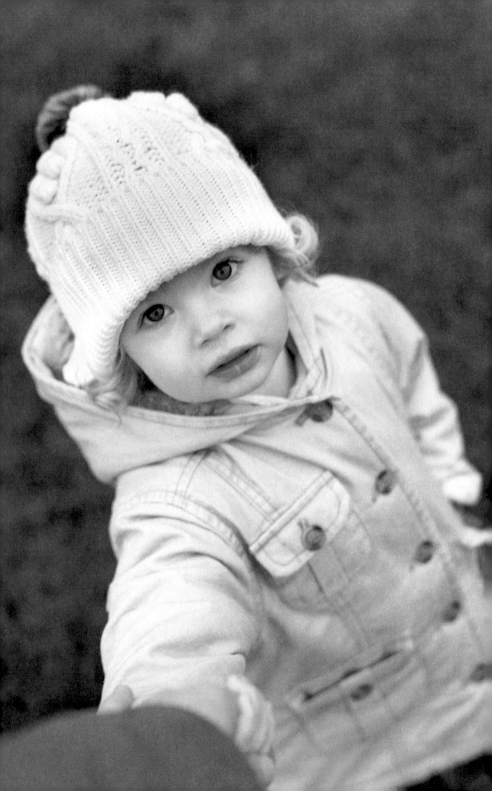

SECOND-TIME MUM

The first morning in hospital, the day after Daisy was born, was very similar to the first morning that I had spent with Poppy just over a year before. I vividly remember lying in my bed facing Daisy in her little plastic crib and feeling that same rush of excitement as I gazed at her. I even had *Trisha* on the TV in the background! I ordered the same breakfast that I had had the previous year (honey on toast with tea and orange juice). But even with all these similarities and familiarities there was something very different about the whole experience. I couldn't quite put my finger on it but it soon became obvious to me that I was 1,000 times more relaxed about the whole thing this time around. I actually ate my breakfast and enjoyed my tea. I even had another pot without checking to see if Daisy was all right in her cradle. I also relaxed while in the shower and didn't panic that I wouldn't be able to hear her cry. And I certainly didn't fuss about with the breastfeeding sheet that I had been given to fill in. No, I was now a confident second-time mum and proud of it too!

It was also a rather strange experience for me not to want to rush home. I was secretly enjoying the pampering I was receiving and the little bit of a lie-in which I had missed so badly since having Poppy. But on the other hand, I was so eager to see Poppy – it was ridiculous that I was missing her so much. I hadn't even been gone 24 hours but it was the longest we had ever been apart and it hurt!

With my mum and Lisa taking care of Poppy at home, I didn't have to worry about her, but they obviously were because it seemed like every five minutes they called me to ask my advice on which outfit she should wear to visit her new sister in hospital (all this must run in the family!).

With great anticipation, Daisy and I awaited the arrival of Princess Pops; I was slightly worried about her reaction. With the video camera at the ready, Jamie, Mum, Lisa and finally, Pops, put their heads round the door. Not yet able to walk, Poppy crawled on to my bed and eyed Daisy suspiciously as she fed at my breast but, as predicted, she soon got bored and was raring to crawl along the hospital corridor!

So that was it. Wow! We thought she didn't seem at all jealous . . . well, until we got home and then I soon started to discover just how difficult it was going to be having to care for a newborn as well as giving full attention to a demanding little 13-month-old.

ONE YEAR ON . . .

I've focused more on Poppy's development throughout the book as little Daisy fit in with our family life and pretty much went through the same routines that I had with Poppy. Having an older sister to look up to and copy, she tended to pick things up quickly. But when it came to eating solids it was a different matter. At first she struggled, so I decided to skip the rice, thinking that she would perhaps prefer some stewed apple – she was six months old at this point. To my disappointment, of Daisy was the complete opposite of Poppy when it came to eating – she couldn't even swallow the apple. I became concerned and started to wonder if she had something wrong with her palate or the roof of her mouth for

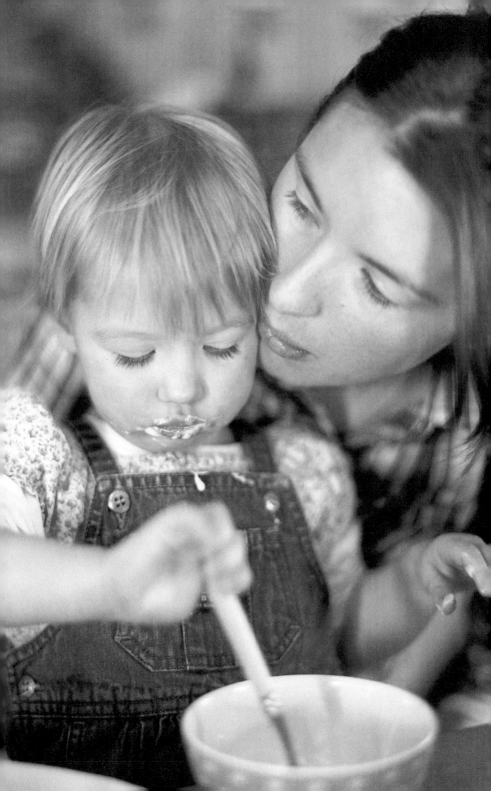

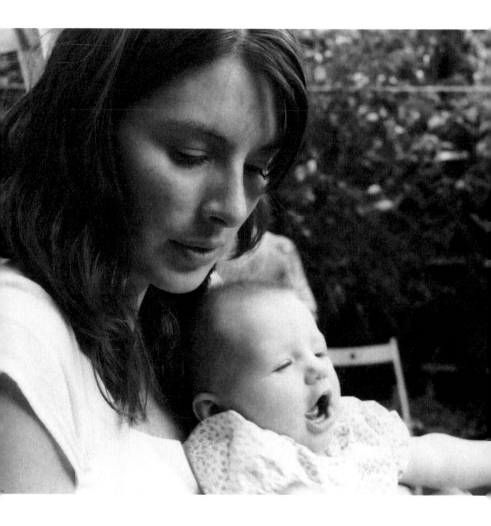

that matter, but all my worrying was unnecessary. Within a month of starting her on solids, she was packing in like the best of them, and still is to this day. Since then she has never refused to eat food and hasn't become a fussy eater. In fact, I only have to open the oven door or set the table and Daisy has learned at 15 months to get herself into her high chair and put on her bib. Surprisingly, she has been feeding herself since she was one . . . astounding. Like father, like daughter!

I soon began to realize that with two children to look after, spending hours at a time cooking is not on the top of the agenda. Other priorities take over. So I stopped doing the cook-offs and freezer sessions so often. Instead, once a month I made up a big fish pie and portioned it off into bags for the freezer, or a Bolognese sauce or a chicken casserole. These freezer foods became my savior if I knew that I would be having a busy week with no time to concentrate on cooking. I always keep some food in the freezer for emergencies.

If I do have time in the day, I simply cook for the girls using fresh ingredients. I mean, I'm talking simple things here. Their favorite meal is fresh salmon with either minty peas or broccoli and grated Parmesan cheese – it's so quick to make, and easy too. Another time-saving trick is to make a tiny bit more to see us over to the next day. So, perhaps with the cooked salmon I would then make them a Jools-style fish pasta with vegetables, which they love, and it only takes minutes. See "The Food Bit" (page 255) where I've included some of the recipes that I make on a regular basis, along with a list of cupboard essentials.

I'm passionate about what goes into my kids' mouths! I know that I am extremely lucky to have the time to give them what I consider the best possible start in life regarding food, and I know that many families might not be able to do this, so I hope that some of my little ideas might help. I most certainly condone jars of baby food – they are an essential when you are on a trip out or when you find yourself with an empty pantry or fridge. However, if you can manage the one big cook-off every now and then it will work out to be far cheaper and, of course, you have the added bonus of knowing exactly which ingredients you are feeding your baby.

I was recently called a Nazi mother by some small-minded journalist in one of the papers! Not only did I find this extremely offensive, but it's also ridiculous. Jamie had mentioned in an interview that I am fanatical about giving my children fresh fruit and that I even take some to children's parties for them to eat. Yes, I *do* do this. I mean, my girls are only 18 months and 2½ years old and if you can't control their eating habits now, then when can you? I am only trying to give them the best possible start in life and I know only too well that when they reach four or five they will be eating chocolate and cakes whether I like it or not. And let me just finish this little rant by saying that, contrary to popular belief, my girls do have treats – and yummy ones at that (just not chocolate buttons like this particular journalist gave her children). So, to each their own, I say. I think us mums have a tough enough job as it is being parents, so it's best not to judge anyone who is obviously trying to do the best for their babies!

BOUNCY TO HIGH . . .
THE CHAIR'S THE THING

Well, the next thing on my agenda regarding feeding habits was when to move Poppy into a high chair. I had already bought one and it was waiting to be assembled, so it was with great excitement that when she seemed able to sit up unaided, I knew she might be ready for her first high chair! It was fantastic and so much easier to feed her at the table, as opposed to me sitting cross-legged on the floor in front of her.

I think I have an obsession with high chairs, as I've managed to get through five different ones in just two years. I view the high chair section in a magazine as avidly and excitedly as Jamie views the cars on *Top Gear* . . . you see it's all about the make and the model and what each one can do. Kids don't know how good they've got it these days! The most important feature for us, though, was whether it could be folded away to maximize space, as our dining room didn't have all that much room around the table. I wasn't keen on the really high-tech plastic supermodel of the high-chair world, as they all seemed to have garish seat colors and huge legs, so we opted for a traditional wooden one – a classic, just like an old Morris Minor! I have now managed to either give my many high chairs away or put them into storage, since we have now graduated on to the toddler chairs, which the girls love. I'm sure it makes them feel more grown up, even with Daisy being just 18 months!

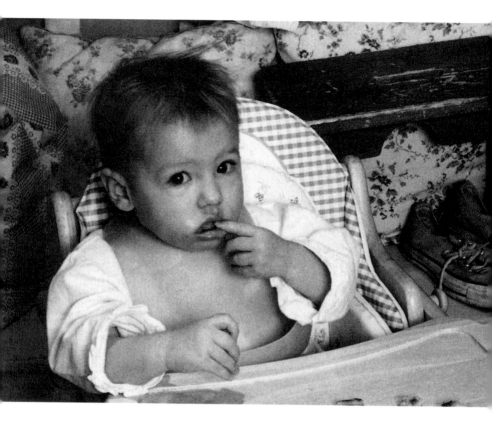

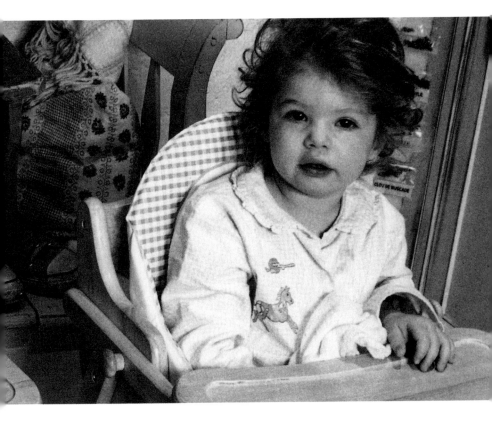

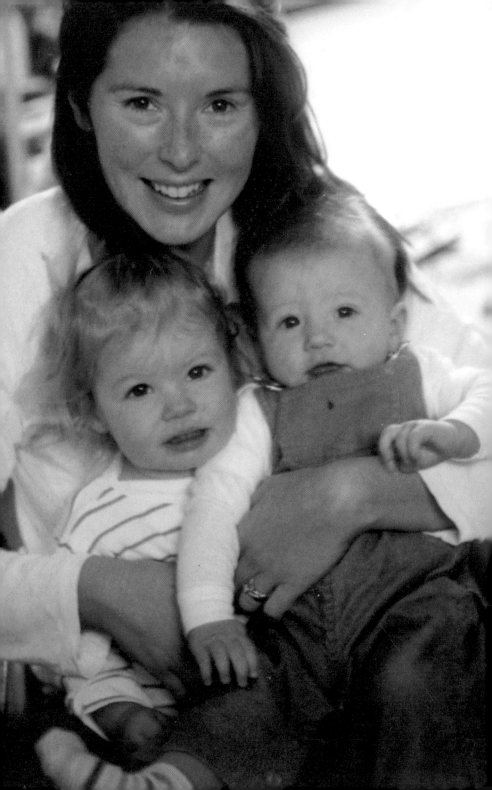

Minus Nine to Two ...
Life with Poppy and Daisy

BECOMING GOOD PARENTS

Jamie and I still have so much to learn when it comes to being good parents. I think we are doing a fine job, but there are definitely times, like today for example, when we had to cope with Poppy lying screaming on the floor of an antiques shop. Not to be left out, Daisy decided to try and buckeroo herself out of the push chair, hysterically gathering up rogue raisins which she'd dropped on her lap and screaming for her blankie which she had lost somewhere along the way. It was one of those moments of hell as we felt completely defeated by their behavior and at a complete loss as to how we should cope with it. We left the shop immediately and cut what was supposed to be a fun day trip short and headed home, stressed, tired and with me close to tears. I think it was just "one of those days" which most parents have to deal with – it's just not much fun when it happens.

When these tantrums started, rather than dragging our perfectly well-adjusted children to a psychiatrist, I decided it was time to get clued in on how to cope with the terrible twos x 2! Here are some of the ways that I try to discipline my two when they misbehave ...

1 The naughty corner

A couple of months ago I started to implement a disciplinary tactic called "the naughty corner." I'd seen this work on a television show about parenting and am pleased to say that it works. It's especially effective at meal times when both girls, but Poppy especially, tend to get fractious and test us, knowing that eating and enjoying your food is something that both Jamie and I find important. The other night she must have made it to the naughty corner three times before she happily sat down and ate her fish! It's simple. All we do is get down to her level and then calmly (which can be hard!) explain that we are not happy with how she is behaving and that she will stay there until she can say sorry and eat her dinner. I always reward her with a gentle voice and a big cuddle and kiss. Honestly, it does the trick. There were a few initial problems – like finding a good place to have as the naughty corner. The first one I chose happened to be where I kept my battered cowboy boots and within a minute I realized that Poppy was quiet because she was trying my boots on and having a great time!

We've just moved into a new house in London and I have yet to nominate a space to act as the "naughty corner." On the spur of the moment, I sat Poppy at the bottom of the stairs going down into the kitchen, only for her to tell me that she was in the wrong corner and that Daddy had put her in the opposite one just the night before! The funny thing is, she does actually stay there for the three minutes or so that I leave her alone. Kids! You can't win sometimes, but you have to stick with it and not give in, back down or laugh (at times this can be very hard, too!).

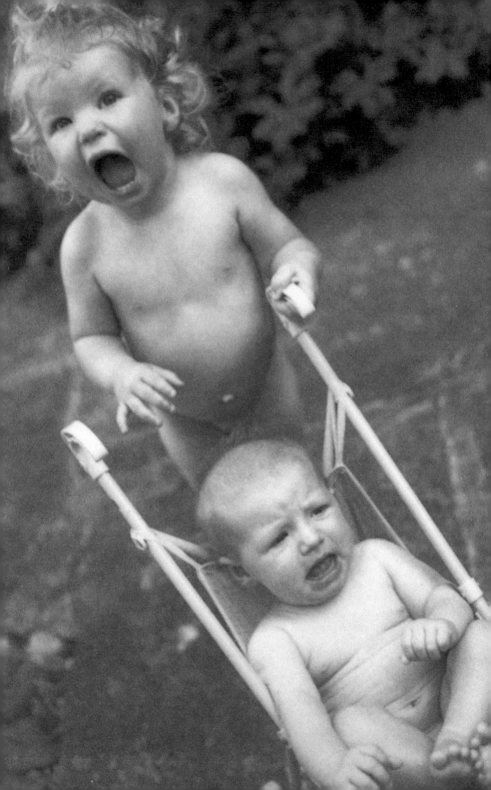

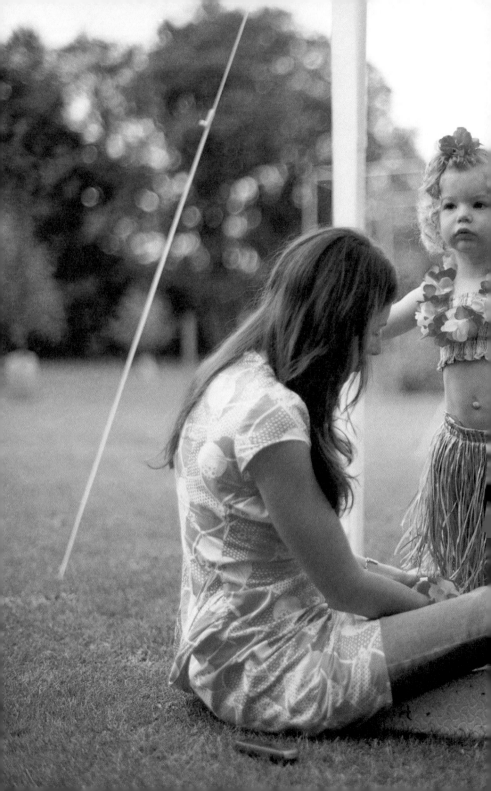

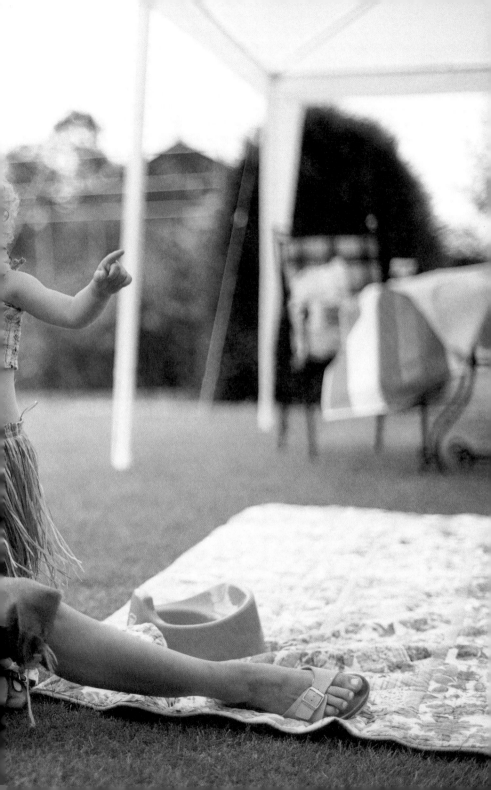

I've come to realize that you can't be inconsistent with your punishments, otherwise the children don't understand if they are doing something they shouldn't. I do find it amazing that at the tender age of 2½, Poppy is well aware of whether she has done something wrong. So much so that if she is in the process of a naughty act, like raiding the pantry or climbing on the table, she will say, "Please go away, Mummy, don't look!"

2 Not shouting

I try never to shout at the girls, but any parent will understand that this is almost impossible at times (unless you have the patience of a saint, which I don't). But I do think that shouting gets in the way of what you are trying to say to them and if that's all they hear then maybe they won't understand what they've done wrong. Instead, I attempt to get eye contact on their level and will say, for example, "Mummy is very angry and you have been very naughty." I think that Poppy knows by listening to me emphasizing those words that I'm not happy with her. Afterward she always wants my affection.

3 Asking advice from family or friends

My sister Nat has been such a fantastic help to me. I really look up to her and take all her advice to heart. Having her there to answer my endless questions has been a huge help. Whether I needed information on silly things like packing a baby's overnight bag, or whether a thermal shirt is needed at night as well as a onesie, she has always been there with her precious advice which I will always hold on to.

My other sister, Lisa, has helped me look after both my

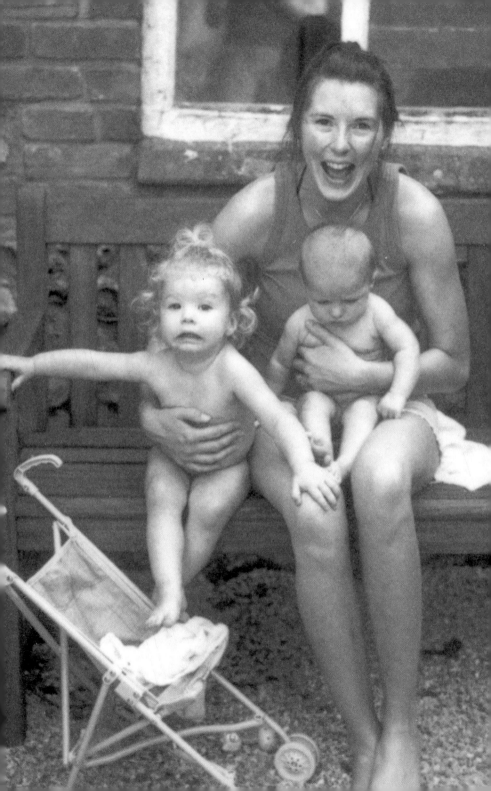

children from the day they were born. She doesn't have children herself, yet she is absolutely fantastic with my two. We have certainly both learned together and now she has ridiculously strong opinions on car seats, push chairs, high chairs, sippy cups . . . you name it! She is going to be a brilliant mum one day.

I realize that every parent has a completely different way of bringing up their children. Although Lisa respects the way that Jamie and I do things, she knows already that she will do things a bit differently by having a more relaxed routine, and that's great. At the end of the day, it's all about what suits you and your lifestyle best.

Jamie and I are definitely still learning, and probably always will be! I worry all the time about whether I'm doing things right or wrong, but I guess there is no particular answer. I think if you give your children the biggest amount of love, affection, warmth, respect and understanding you can't go far wrong.

MOMENTS AND MILESTONES

For all the tantrums, there are double the amount of great moments and that is what makes being a parent all worth it. I remember when Poppy grabbed her bottle of milk from me one morning and lay there feeding herself. I was so shocked at this big move to independence, as well as being immensely impressed and excited. It was at that point that I decided to encourage her to use a spoon and fork – do it for Mummy! But I suppose that is just human nature. No sooner had Poppy shown signs of crawling than I was out

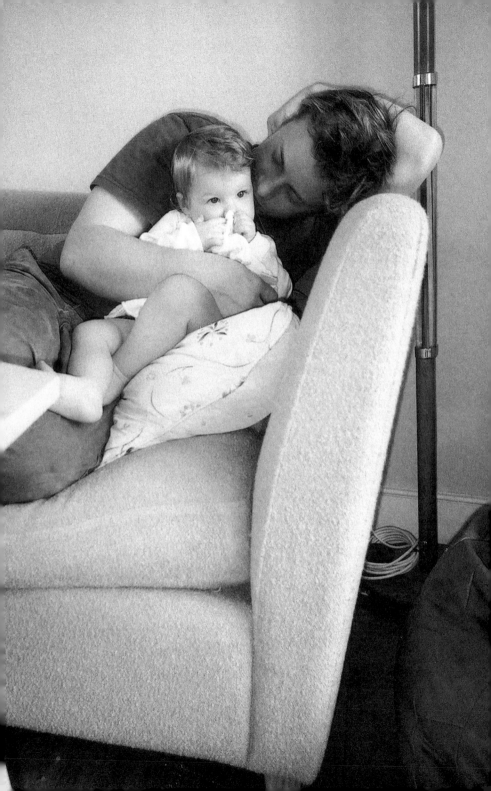

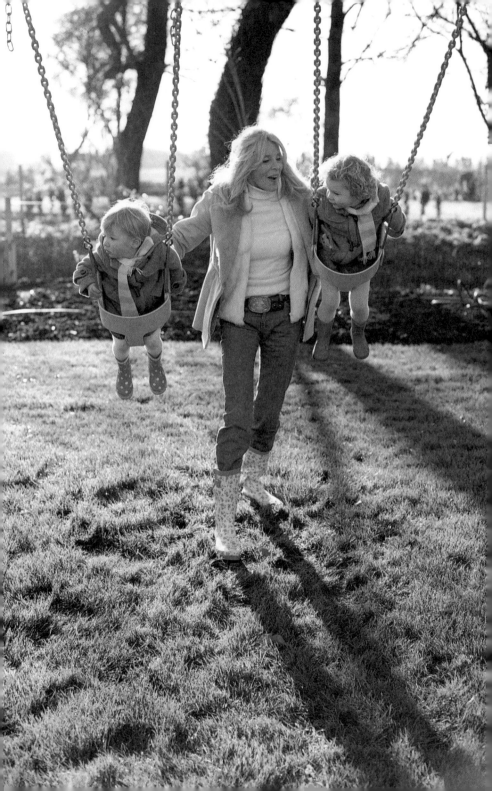

buying her first pair of walking shoes! But it was a long while before that happened. She spent the best part of $2^1/_2$ months dragging herself along the wooden floors in our house like a snake, using only her elbows to gather momentum and speed. It was great to watch her, especially when we realized that she looked like a soldier on an assault mission! But with plenty of encouragement and coaching from Jamie, it wasn't long before she was able to pull herself up on the furniture and cruise around the room from piece to piece.

Although I knew I should just savor the moment, I did want to rush this stage of development as I so wanted to see her take her first dash through the leaves in her wellies. All too soon that dream became a reality when Poppy was 13 months and Daisy was only two weeks old. We had some friends over for a glass of wine one evening and as they cooed over our beautiful newborn, Poppy obviously felt left out, so she leapt up from drinking her milk and walked across the room! Now, I'd read that your child's first step is exciting but for us that was an understatement. It really takes a lot to beat that moment of seeing her proud face as she triumphantly strode across the room from one of our friends to the another. Luckily Jamie had managed to witness it. As he works so hard I was convinced that he would miss all the milestones that our babies would reach, but there he was with tears in his eyes videotaping the whole thing.

I know it's hard, but try not to will your baby's next stage to hurry up. There are times now when I wish Poppy was that little crawling commando soldier clinging on to my feet instead of a tear-away terrible two (but a cute one at that!). As my mum-in-law once told me, "It is better to travel hopefully than to arrive."

One of the huge milestones I was really looking forward to was Poppy's first birthday. I was most concerned that I would be huffing and puffing to push baby number two out instead of helping Poppy to blow out her first birthday candle! But Daisy had other ideas and, not wanting to steal Poppy's thunder, she decided that it would be best to stay inside me way past her due date! Poppy's first birthday was lovely. Jamie managed to get the day off work and the three (well, four!) of us spent the morning in the park and the afternoon at the zoo. I am not sure that she was aware of it being a special day but we loved it. Jamie had baked her a cake and cooked a fish pie. I love watching the video and can't believe how huge I was when carrying Daisy. Just a year later we were celebrating Daisy's first birthday in exactly the same tradition – park, zoo, cake (but this time I made it – a rather classic Victoria sponge with a bunny rabbit on the top – in fact, it was better than the one Jamie had made the year before!). We bought Daisy the same 1st birthday present that we got for Poppy – a beautiful blossom tree standing only a couple of feet high against Poppy's six-footer. It is just a small reminder to Jamie and me how far we have all come as a family and how we continue to grow.

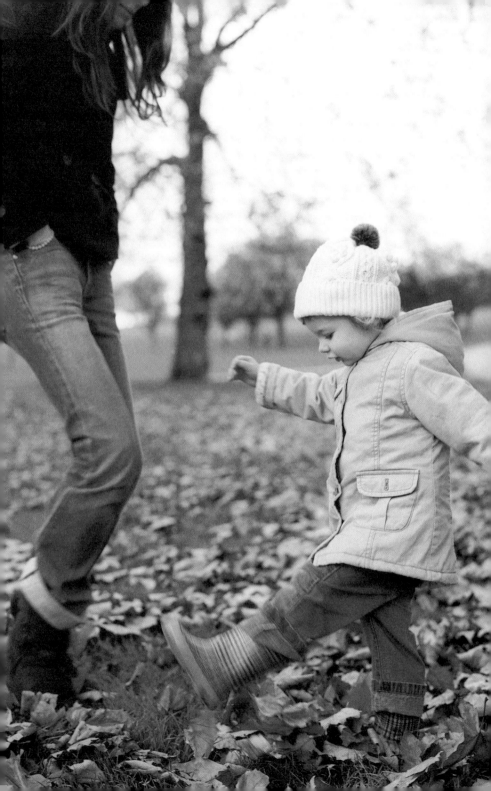

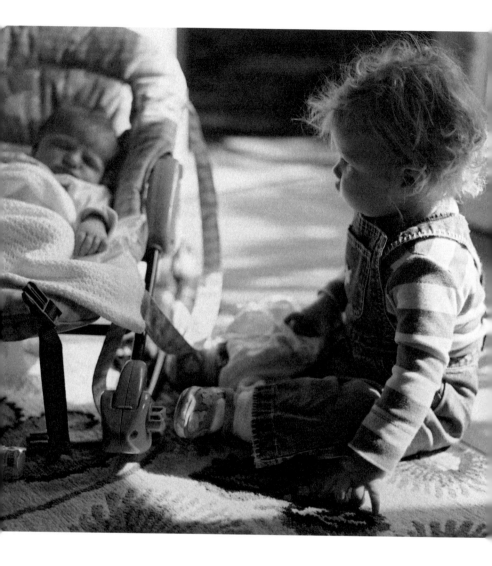

SISTERS

When I think back now to when Daisy was newborn, I can't help but laugh. Jamie and I were so concerned that Poppy shouldn't feel jealous. Every morning Jamie would bring Poppy downstairs to have her usual bottle of milk in our bed and every morning, without fail, she would peep her little blonde curly head around our bedroom door and give a look of horror as she realized that Daisy was still there. Her bottom lip would stick out in a great big pout as she watched Daisy feeding. I really don't think that she could get her little head around it!

After a while, and a few instances of tackling, pinching and over-cuddling and the odd prod of the Moses basket, Poppy finally realized that Daisy was here to stay.

It was, and still is at times, hard work to have had two babies so close to each other. In the beginning, if I wasn't changing Pop's nappy then it was Daisy's. I had Daisy permanently attached to me like a little limpet in case Poppy might accidentally hurt her. Now I constantly find myself battling with them over sharing their books and the ballerina doll that they both HAVE to have at the same time even though I bought one for each of them. I dread to think what they might be like as teenagers – the arguments we will have over makeup!

A lot of people say to me that it's worth having children close together to "get it over and done with and out of the way," but I hate that saying. I never wanted to get my pregnancies and babies rushed through like groceries at a

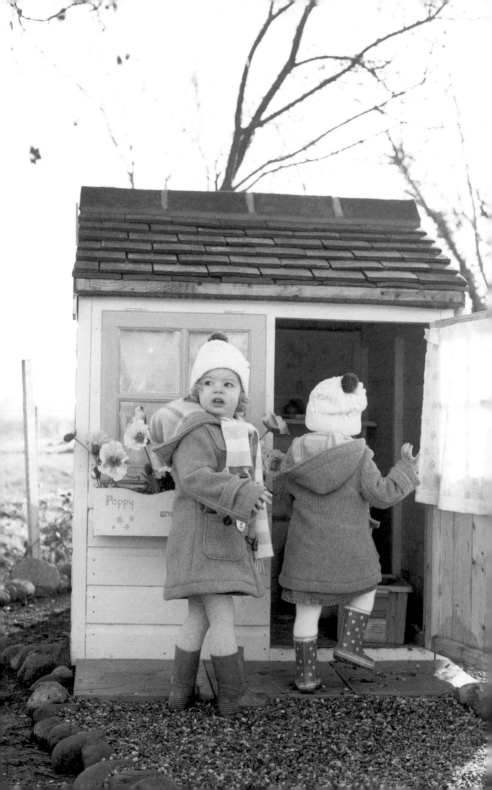

supermarket checkout. Jamie and I really wanted to devour each experience and enjoy each child. That perhaps would have been our only criticism about the experience; we worried that each child was not getting the level of attention which they both so deserved, but I believe that it has been great for the girls to have each other there as they are now so close.

As the months have passed, Daisy has become less of a toy for Poppy and more of a mini-friend. We often catch little glimpses of Poppy stealing a sneaky kiss or putting her arm around Daisy while they are watching *Noddy* from their high chairs. I find it so fascinating to watch them play together. Unlike what I expected, Daisy is the definite leader while Pops follows behind. She copies everything that Daisy does – from silly noises to funny dance moves – and she always looks to us for the ultimate approval. Whereas Daisy couldn't care less about what Jamie and I think – as long as she is having a good time! In many ways they are like chalk and cheese, from Daisy's dead straight hair to Poppy's goldilocks curls.

When I am reading to them at night and they are sitting there holding hands, it reminds me so much of how I was with my two sisters. The three of us are very close now, and so it is these moments that make me really happy. Although she was a very unexpected surprise, I'm so glad that Daisy came along to join us when she did. Now it's time to look forward to any future additions to our family!

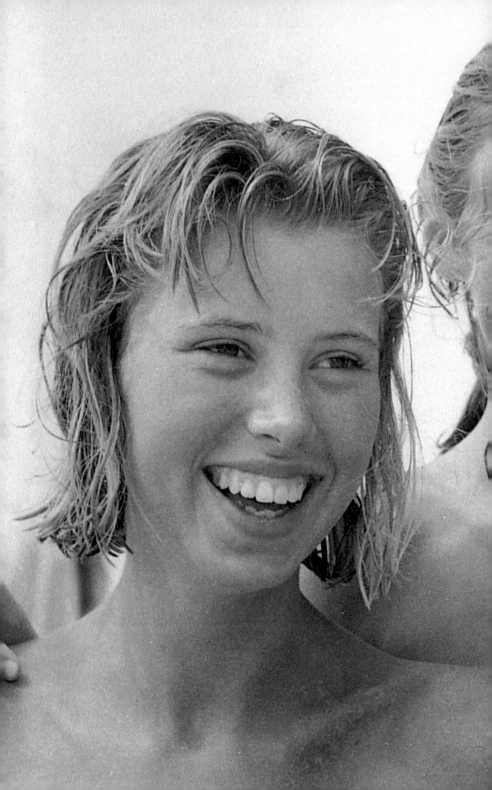

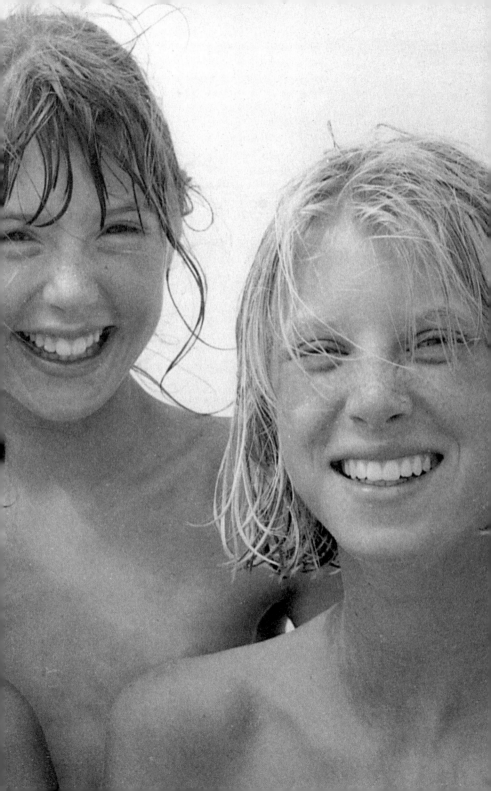

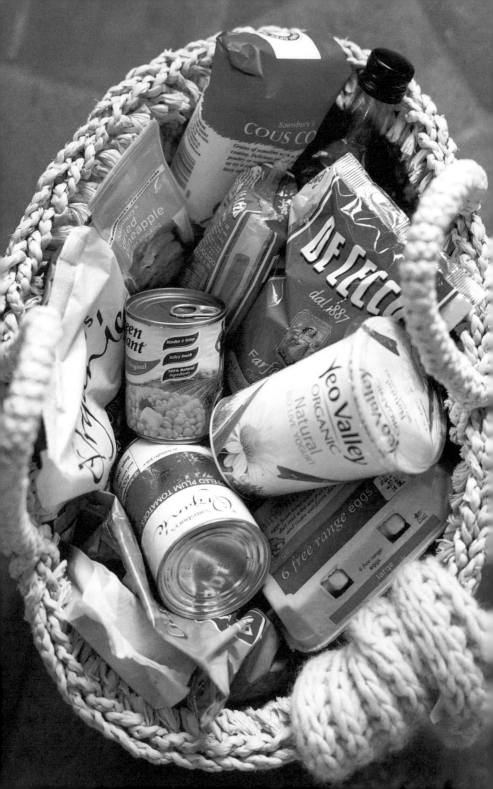

The Food Bit

Cupboard essentials

When it comes to feeding the girls, I always make sure that I have the following list of things in the cupboard, fridge or freezer. This way I can decide whether to buy some fish or chicken, and can stock up on fresh fruit and vegetables every couple of days.

* Cans of plum tomatoes
* Cans of salt- and sugar-free sweet corn
* Frozen peas
* Parmesan or Cheddar cheese
* Eggs
* Small pasta shapes (like fusillini, which are little twists, or conchiglette, which are little shells)
* Rice
* Couscous
* Organic oats
* Dried fruit
* Natural yogurt

Equipment
* Freezer bags
* Ice-cube trays
* Hand blender
* Food processor
* Sieve

RECIPES

Here are a few of the recipes which I make on a regular basis for the girls. The emphasis is on ease and quickness!

FRUIT SMOOTHIE

This is a great one to do if you can't get your child to eat fruit. You can choose all different types of fruit to mix together – it's a great way of using up older fruit but you can also freeze your fruit once it's ripe and then peel it, chop it up and then put it straight in the blender for a really cold refreshing drink. The oatmeal is there to give added goodness and to make it lovely and creamy. I usually make more than I need and then I keep it in the fridge for the next day. You will need to have a blender to make this.

MAKES 6 SERVINGS
1 banana, peeled
1 papaya, peeled, halved and seeded
1 mango, peeled and pitted
1 kiwi, peeled
1/2 cup old-fashioned rolled oats
1 x 1-pound of natural plain yogurt
a few ice cubes (if your fruit is not frozen)

Put all your prepared fruit in a blender with the rolled oats, yogurt and ice cubes and blitz until smooth.

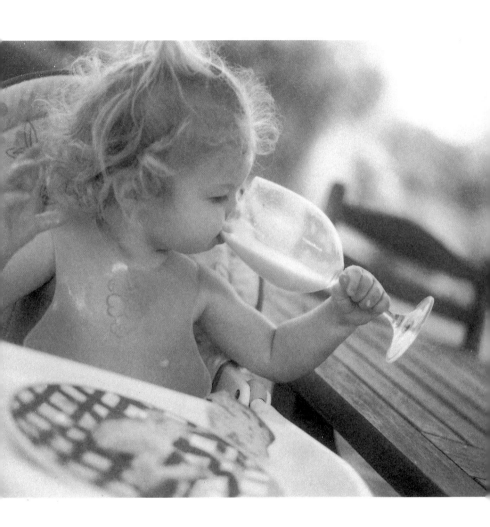

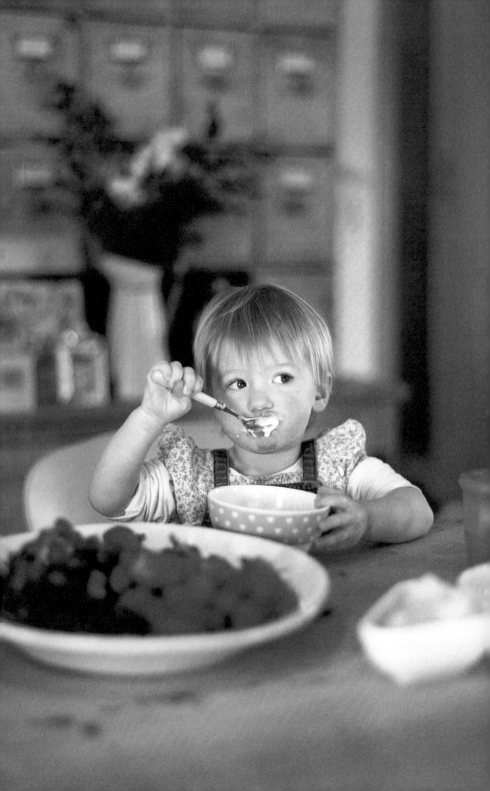

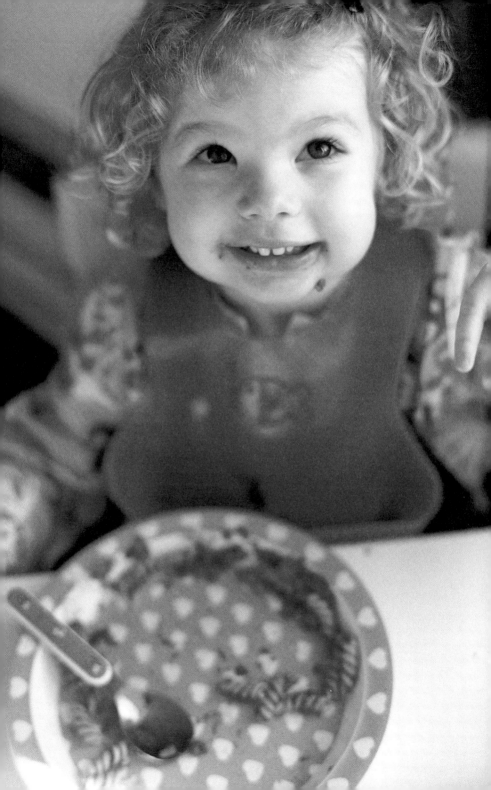

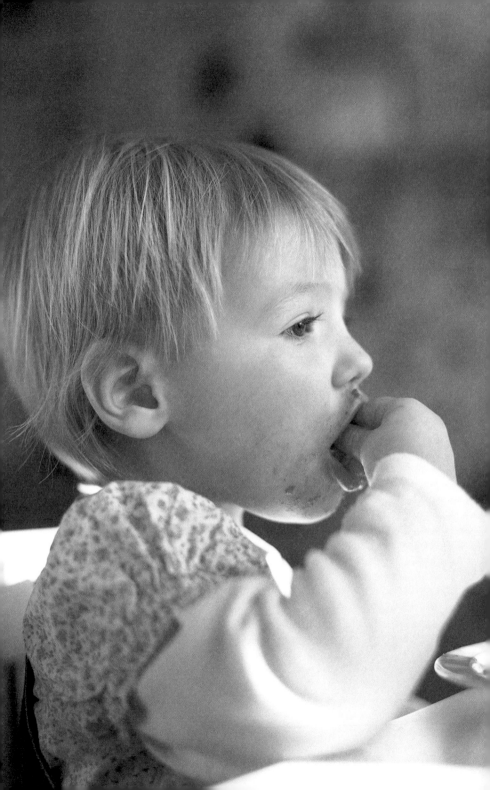

ROASTED BUTTERNUT SQUASH WITH MINT, CRÈME FRAÎCHE AND PASTA

This is fantastically easy to make – all you need to do is pop it in the oven for about an hour and a half. If you only want enough for one or two children, then cook a couple of portions of pasta and mix with two spoonfuls of the roasted, mashed squash. The rest of the squash can be frozen in ice-cube trays to give instant small portions.

MAKES 8 SERVINGS

1 butternut squash
2 cups (about 7 ounces) small pasta shapes (see Cupboard
     Essentials list for varieties)
2 tablespoons crème fraîche
a small handful of fresh mint leaves, finely chopped

Preheat the oven to 350°F. Wrap the squash in aluminum foil and place directly on an oven rack, then roast it for 1½ hours. When the squash is cooked, put a pot of water on to boil and then add your pasta to it. It should only need 6–8 minutes, but check the package instructions. Take the slightly cooled butternut squash, halve it, remove the seeds and scoop out all the lovely orange squash. Roughly mash or chop the squash and then mix it with your cooked and drained pasta. Dollop some crème fraîche on the top and stir through to make a creamy sauce. Sprinkle with some finely chopped mint.

BOLOGNESE

This is always a good one as children tend to love the taste and they find it easy to eat. It's also a great way to give them vegetables as you can chop and change what you use depending on the season. I've recently started adding sweet potato to mine and the girls love it. The bacon adds a nice sweetness. When I make bolognese I usually make up a big batch and then divide it into small freezer bags. This way you can take one out of the freezer the night before you need it and leave it to defrost in the fridge. It can then be heated up quickly. I serve it either on its own with some finely grated Parmesan cheese over the top or mixed with some cooked and drained little pasta shapes.

MAKES 10–15 SERVINGS
olive oil
4 slices streaky bacon or pancetta
1/2 a leek, trimmed and diced
1 clove of garlic, peeled and finely chopped
1 carrot, peeled and diced
1 stick of celery, trimmed and diced
1 small zucchini, diced
1/2 a red pepper, seeded and diced
1 small sweet potato, peeled and grated or finely chopped
1 handful of mushrooms, chopped
1 pound lean ground beef
1 sprig fresh rosemary or thyme
1 bay leaf
1 28-once can of plum tomatoes
(optional) 1/2 15.5 ounce can of chickpeas

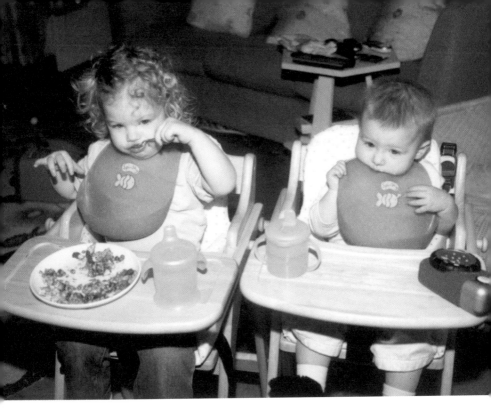

Put a deep saucepan on a medium heat. Add a splash of olive oil,
the bacon, the leek and the garlic. Cook for 5 minutes, stirring, and
then add the rest of the vegetables and cook for 5 minutes more.
Now add your meat, herbs (the bay leaf and herb sprig can be put in
whole and removed at the end), tomatoes, chickpeas and a chickpea
can full of water. Allow to simmer slowly for 1 hour. Remember to
remove the herbs before serving.

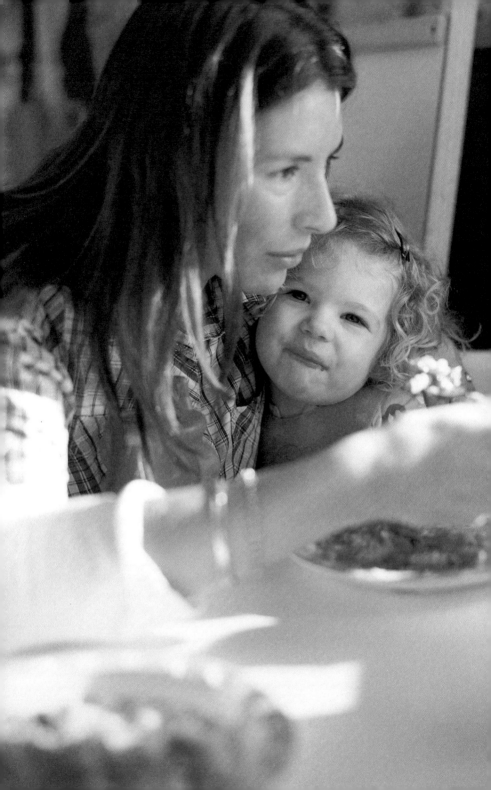

CHICKEN CASSEROLE

This is very simple and very tasty – don't worry about the garlic being too strong as the long cooking time means the taste will mellow. I'm quite a big fan of dried herbs, especially when I'm in a rush, but it's also lovely to use fresh chopped parsley or thyme if you have some on hand.

MAKES 8–10 SERVINGS

2 whole, boneless chicken breasts, skin removed
2 cloves of garlic, peeled and halved
1/2 teaspoon dried mixed herbs
finely ground black pepper
1 1/4 cups of canned chicken broth, or the same
    amount of broth made with a bouillon cube
2 parsnips, peeled and roughly chopped
2 carrots, peeled and roughly chopped
1/2 a small rutabaga, peeled and roughly chopped
4 medium potatoes, peeled and roughly chopped
1 leek, cleaned and roughly chopped
1 stick of celery

Preheat the oven to 400°F. Put the chicken breasts in a casserole dish with the garlic. Sprinkle the dried mixed herbs over the chicken, with a grinding of black pepper. Pour in the chicken stock, add your chopped vegetables and then top up with water so that everything is covered. Put the casserole dish in the oven for 1 1/2 hours. When cooked, remove it from the oven and allow it to cool before mashing it all up. (You will have to remove the bone from the chicken breasts.) I either use an egg beater or a fork (the texture will obviously depend on how old your baby is). For Poppy I usually cut it up for her, whereas Daisy will have it mashed. A great one to freeze in little freezer bags.

CHICKEN AND RICE WITH VEGETABLES

This is a great recipe for using up leftover chicken from your Sunday roast, or you can roast off a fresh breast. It's also easy to turn this into a fish dish, by substituting the chicken with a white fish fillet. It's important to remember that any uneaten bits are thrown away and not put in the freezer as you're using previously cooked food. However, if you decide to make it using fresh ingredients, then you can freeze any leftovers.

MAKES 4–6 SERVINGS

1 handful of shredded cooked chicken or 1 fresh whole boneless
    chicken breast
1 14-ounce can of plum tomatoes
3 handfuls or $1/4$ uncooked basmati rice
2 handfuls of fresh and prepared or leftover cooked veggies
    (try 1 ounce broccoli, $1/2$ a 15.5-ounce can of sweet corn, 1 ounce
peas or 2 ounces spinach)

Preheat the oven to 350°F. Put your leftover shredded chicken breast or your whole chicken breast into an ovenproof saucepan. Add your tomatoes, the rice and a little cold water. If your vegetables are uncooked, add them now. Put the pan on the burner and bring to the boil, then transfer it to the oven for 12–15 minutes until the rice is all nice and fluffy. If you are using leftover vegetables, then pop them into the saucepan 5 minutes before the end of the cooking time.

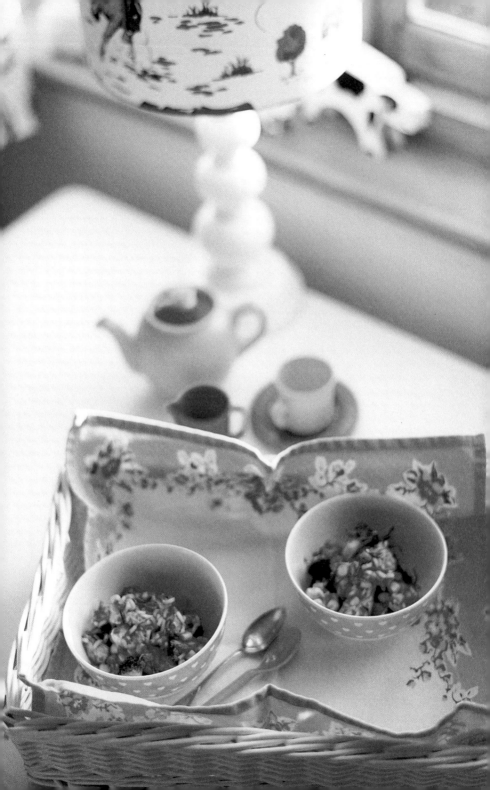

LEMON BUTTERED PLAICE

Plaice fillets, also called fluke, are really thin so you don't have to mash the fish too much when it's cooked. One whole plaice fillet can feed two children. I usually ask my fishmonger to fillet and skin my fish. The great thing about this recipe is that you can add sweet corn (no added salt or sugar), peas or spinach and mash it all up together.

MAKES 2 SERVINGS
1 sweet potato
1 small fillet of plaice, fluke, or flounder
juice of $1/2$ a lemon
a pat of butter
a sprinkling of mixed dried herbs or use a little fresh,
    chopped flat-leaf parsley or basil
olive oil

Wrap the sweet potato in aluminum foil and put it in the oven at 300°F for an hour or so (good if you need to run an errand!), then remove it and keep it warm. Turn the oven up to 400°F. Place the fish fillet in a baking pan. Squeeze over the lemon juice and put the butter on top. Sprinkle with some dried herbs and drizzle with a little olive oil. Place in the oven for 8–10 minutes. Scoop out the orange flesh of the potato, remove the fish from the oven and either whip or mash up – brilliant food for toddlers and babies.

PLAICE IN TOMATO SAUCE

This is such an easy dish to prepare, and is so good for children.
You can replace the fish fillet with a chicken breast if you like.
Just cook it for an extra 10–12 minutes until cooked through.
Shred or cut into little pieces before serving.

MAKES 2 SERVINGS

3/4 cup crushed tomatoes
1 small fillet of plaice, fluke, flounder or other white fish
a small handful of fresh basil leaves, picked and chopped
a small handful of freshly grated Parmesan or Cheddar cheese
olive oil

Preheat the oven to 400°F. Pour your tomatoes into a small
ovenproof dish and place your fish fillet on top. Sprinkle with the
chopped basil and grated cheese and drizzle over a little olive oil. Pop
the dish into the oven for 8–10 minutes. When the fish is cooked,
flake it with a fork and mix it into the tomato sauce. This is great with
mashed or baked potatoes.

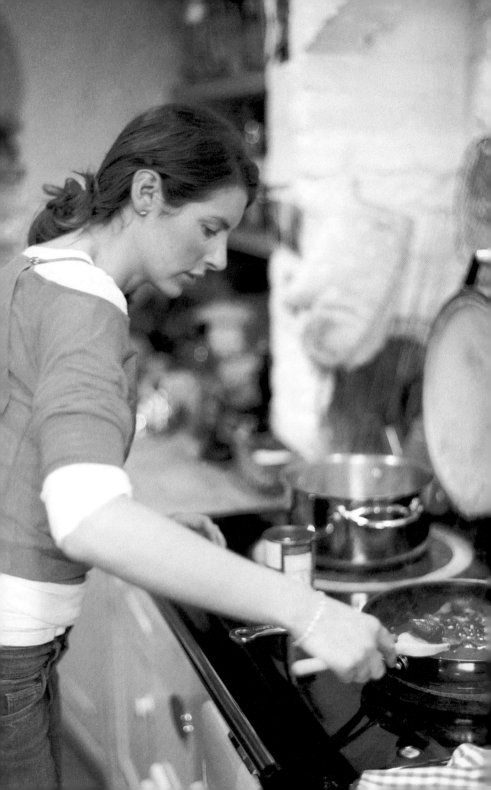

SALMON WITH BROCCOLI AND ORANGE

The fruitiness of the orange in this dish really sweetens up the fish.
Salmon is a great fish to include in your baby's diet, as it contains
omega-3 oil, which is good for brain and memory. This can be served
with some mashed-up leftover potatoes or some cooked and
drained little pasta shapes.

MAKES 2 SERVINGS
1 salmon fillet, skinned
1 orange, zest peeled off in strips, juiced
a pat of butter
a handful or 2 ounces little broccoli florets

Preheat your oven to 400°F. Lay a large piece of aluminum foil on a
baking pan and place your salmon on the foil. Squeeze over the
orange juice, place your strips of orange zest on top, with the butter,
and scatter over the broccoli florets. Wrap the foil around the fish in a
parcel and place the pan in the oven for 10–12 minutes.

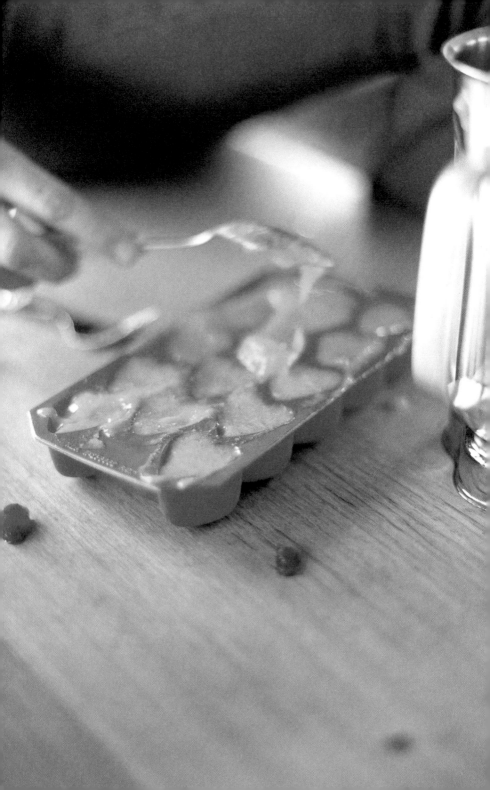

FRESH FRUIT

When it comes to making desserts, there is nothing easier or more full of goodness than fresh fruit with yogurt. If you introduce it early on, then your child will hopefully grow to love fruit. Poppy thinks that mango pieces are sweets, and having a little bowl of blueberries is a treat for her. She also loves strawberries cut up into bite-sized pieces. I try to give her and Daisy a whole mixture of interesting-looking fruit.

STEWED FRUIT

This is so easy to make and it can be stored in the fridge for a few days, or frozen in ice-cube trays. It's great with either a dollop of natural yogurt or some vanilla ice cream as a treat!

SOME LOVELY COMBINATIONS ARE:

❖ Blackberry and apple – 2 Bramley apples, peeled, halved and cored; a handful of blackberries
❖ Rhubarb and ginger – 1 1/2 pounds (approximately 5 sticks) rhubarb, roughly chopped; a thumb-sized piece of ginger, grated
❖ Strawberry and pear – 3 pears, peeled, halved and cored; a handful of strawberries
❖ Apricot and vanilla – 1 pound apricots, pitted; 1 vanilla bean, halved and seeds removed

Place your chosen fruit in a saucepan with a couple of tablespoons of water (for the apricots and vanilla, put the bean into the pan as well as the seeds, but remember to remove it before serving or freezing). Cook on a low heat for 10–15 minutes. Once stewed, give it a taste for sweetness. It really depends on the sweetness of your fruit but the rhubarb and ginger, and the apricots and vanilla, will usually benefit from a little added sugar, whereas the strawberry and pear won't need any. Unrefined raw sugar is the best to use.

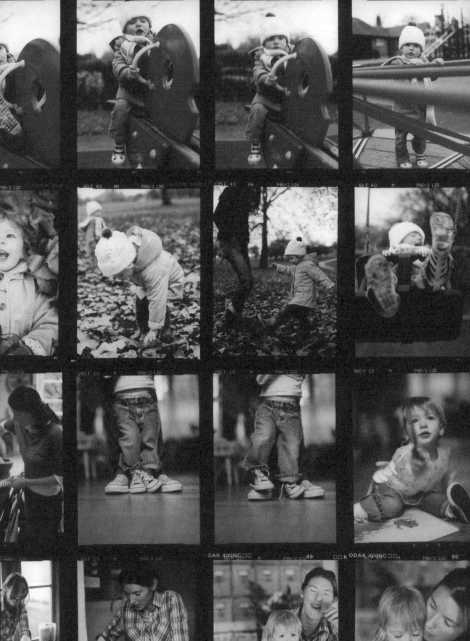

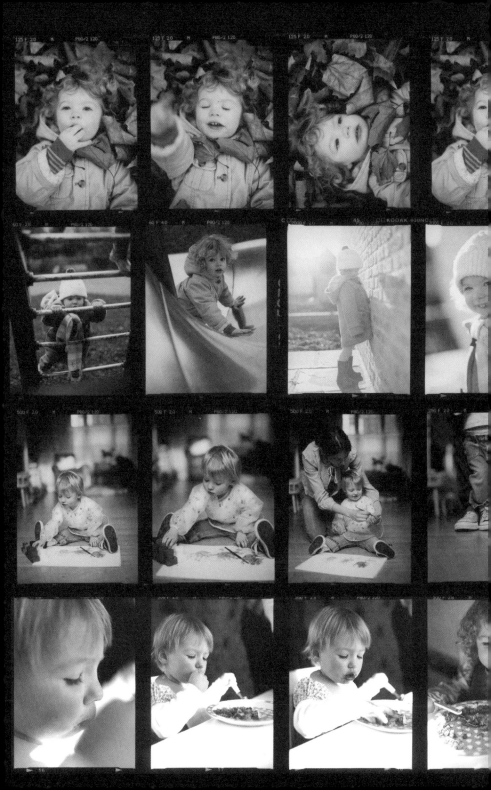

Glossary of Terms

This glossary is intended as a quick reference guide. If you have
any queries or questions after reading it, then a list of helpful
websites (where this information came from) can be found
on page 293, or talk to your community midwife or doctor.

PRE-CONCEPTION

Clomid (clomiphene citrate)
Clomid is a drug that is used to treat infertility when women have
problems ovulating. It is available in tablets. Side effects include
headaches, abdominal discomfort, depression, panic attacks,
hot flushes, nausea, vomiting, convulsions, visual disturbances,
dizziness and insomnia, breast tenderness, weight gain, rashes
and hair loss.

Folic acid
Folic acid is a form of vitamin B that helps prevent a neural tube birth
defect called spina bifida in your baby. You need extra folic acid from
the time you start trying to conceive until the 12th week of pregnancy.
Even if you didn't take folic acid before conceiving, it's worth starting
as soon as you find out you're pregnant. Doctors recommend you
take 0.4 milligram of folic acid every day.

Laparoscopy
Laparoscopy is a visual examination of the inside of the abdomen. A
viewing device is passed through a small cut in the abdominal wall.
Laparoscopy is used by gynecologists to investigate disorders of
the female reproductive organs.

Polycystic ovaries

Polycystic ovary syndrome (PCOS) means that the ovaries, the organs that produce eggs in the female reproductive system, are enlarged and have several fluid-filled sacs or cysts. Women with PCOS may experience a number of other symptoms such as infrequent or no menstrual periods, infrequent or no ovulation, inability to get pregnant within 6 to 12 months of unprotected sexual intercourse (infertility) and diabetes. PCOS is a known cause of infertility and is the most common reproductive problem in women who have ovulation problems. An estimated 5 to 10 percent of women of childbearing age have PCOS (ages 20–40).

FIRST TRIMESTER

Blood tests

In the first trimester, you will most likely be offered a blood test. One sample will be taken to test for the following: your blood group (A, B, O or AB); your Rhesus status; your blood count to rule out conditions like anemia; your blood sugar level to test for diabetes, rubella, syphilis, Hepatitis B and HIV.

Depending on the area in which you live, after 15 weeks of pregnancy you may be offered another blood test which can be used to calculate the chance of Downs syndrome, spina bifida and other neural tube defects. Downs syndrome can also be checked during a **nuchal scan**.

Why do you get the following when pregnant?

Sore boobs: Swollen, tender breasts during pregnancy are caused by the increased amounts of hormones (estrogen and progesterone) being produced in your body. The breast changes are preparing you for breastfeeding later on.

Tiredness: There are lots of reasons in pregnancy for feeling more tired than usual, especially in the first trimester when your body is busy transforming a single cell into a miniature baby, and the last trimester when your baby is active and growing rapidly. To name a few: you are carrying extra weight, your body is working much harder than before, your heart is pumping more blood at a faster rate, your breathing rate has increased and you worry lots more!

Morning sickness/nausea: A feeling of nausea, accompanied by actual sickness in pregnancy, is especially common in the first trimester and is one of the many first signs of pregnancy. It can strike at any time of the day but is more commonly experienced in the morning upon getting out of bed; hence the term "morning" sickness. Although it is very common, some women may sail through pregnancy with no nausea at all. The feeling generally tends to taper off by the 12th week and may even disappear after that. Morning sickness is believed to be associated with the high levels of the pregnancy hormone HCG (Human Chorionic Gonadotrophin), especially in the first trimester.

Food cravings and other weird cravings: It is common in pregnancy to suddenly develop a strong liking for certain foods, as strange as a medley of pickled onions and ice cream. It is great if you develop a craving for nutritious food! However, if the craving is for something fattening and not easily digestible, it is advisable to exercise some control. Remember not to give in to your craving at the expense of a nutritious diet.

A condition in which you crave inedible stuff like coal or soap is called pica and may be due to a nutritional deficiency. It needs to be reported to the doctor or midwife just in case the substance you are craving is dangerous.

Heightened sense of smell: Many women report an altered sensitivity to smell while pregnant. Experts believe that this is caused by the hormonal changes in pregnancy. A heightened sense of smell could be an advantage for pregnant women. Smell is crucial to mother–infant bonding in the first few days following birth. A mother can often tell her own child merely by its smell after a few days.

A need to pee all the time – especially at night! In the first trimester, frequent urination is caused by an increase in the volume of body fluids combined with increased efficiency of the kidneys. In later pregnancy, it is caused by the pressure of the growing uterus and baby on the bladder.

Heartburn: Normally, the sphincter between the food pipe (esophagus) and the stomach prevents stomach acids from passing back into the esophagus. In pregnancy, however, high levels of the hormone progesterone cause it to relax. As a result, the stomach acids pass into the esophagus and irritate its lining. This produces a strong burning sensation in the center of the chest, just where the heart is and hence the term heartburn (although it has nothing to do with the heart).

SECOND TRIMESTER

Colostrum
In mid to late pregnancy, some women experience leakage from their breasts. This is not breast milk but a premilk called colostrum. Actual breast milk is not produced until about three or four days after the delivery. This colostrum leaks as a yellow fluid and may form a crust on the nipples.

Underwire bras

The rigid supports in an underwire bra may interfere with the natural changes in size and shape of the breasts during pregnancy. This can obstruct the increased blood flow, or "squash" the developing milk duct system, causing pain, discomfort and possibly mastitis.

Paracetamol/Tylenol

Tylenol (Acetaminophen) is the safest of all painkillers for use during pregnancy. However, it should be used in moderation and it is always best to ask your midwife or OB for advice.

Bleeding during pregnancy

In the early stages of pregnancy it's quite common to have "spotting," but any bleeding that you experience during your pregnancy must be taken seriously, especially if it occurs during the later stages. If this happens, or you experience severe pelvic pain, the Bounty website (www.bounty.com) recommends that you: contact your doctor, midwife or the hospital labor ward immediately, then either go to bed or find somewhere to rest until help comes, keep hold of any bloodstained clothes and don't flush away blood clots until the doctor or midwife has seen you.

SCANS

What to expect from your 12-week and 20-week scans

Most women will be offered two ultrasound scans during their pregnancy. An ultrasound scan shows your baby and its movements on screen. The first one is usually offered between 10 and 16 weeks, which is about the earliest that any problem can be detected. The baby's development, the due date and the number of babies in your womb may be checked, a **nuchal scan** may be made and any major abnormalities detected. A more detailed check will be done at 18–20 weeks, when the baby's physique, the position of the placenta and the blood flow to the womb are checked.

Doppler scan

A Doppler scan is a special type of ultrasound scan used to examine the flow of blood in the baby or the placenta. It can be used to check for a variety of conditions but is generally only used to scan high-risk women early in pregnancy.

Nuchal scan

The nuchal scan (or the nuchal translucency scan) is not always routine – it depends on where you live – but you can choose to pay privately for one. It is used to measure the nuchal fold at the back of the baby's neck. It is thought that babies with a particularly thick nuchal pad at the back of the neck are at a higher risk of suffering from heart defects, Downs syndrome and other chromosomal abnormalities. Once the risk factor is calculated using this scan, you might be offered a subsequent amniocentesis or other invasive test to confirm, or rule out, these suspicions. The risk of Downs syndrome can also be calculated with a **blood test**.

INDUCING LABOR

If the baby is doing well (prenatal care provided by your midwife or doctor will monitor this), doctors will wait for 41–42 weeks before they induce. In some cases, if the cervix is found to be ripe and ready for delivery, labor may be induced before 42 weeks are up. In cases where the baby is distressed, a caesarean may be carried out to prevent any danger to the baby. Although the preferences of the mother should be the central focus of care, a lot depends on the hospital's policy. Labor can be induced with a **stretch and sweep**, by inserting a **pessary**; through **artificial rupture of membranes** or by administering **syntocinon** (oxytocin).

Artificial rupture of membranes (ARM)

Also called breaking of water, this is an effective way of inducing labor if the cervix is not sufficiently ripe. You will be examined internally by a doctor or midwife and your water will then be broken using an amniohook, which looks like a long, thin plastic crochet hook. Once the membranes are broken, the increased pressure on the cervix causes contractions to become much stronger.

The procedure is painless and is successful in starting labor in the majority of the cases. Once waters are broken, mobility may be restricted, especially if the next step is to add **syntocinon** to your drip.

Induction

A tablet made of prostaglandins is inserted in your vagina. If the cervix is ripe, the pessary stimulates uterine contractions. If the cervix is not ripe, the pessary will help soften the cervix and open it to the extent that at least **ARM** can be carried out. The procedure of placing pessaries in your vagina may be repeated several times during the day until a result is achieved. Sometimes, gel may be used in place of pessaries. This method alone is often not enough to induce labor and is usually combined with **ARM** or **syntocinon**.

Stretch and sweep

A "stretch and sweep" is a way to induce labor. About half of
the women who have this done will naturally go into labor within
48 hours. Your midwife or doctor will do an internal exam and
try to sweep their finger around inside the cervix and loosen the
membranes. It will not increase the risks of infection but it may
feel uncomfortable and you may notice some bleeding. It can be
done at home by your community midwife, in the hospital or at your
prenatal clinic appointment (you can go home afterward
to wait for labor to begin).

Syntocinon (oxytocin)

This is a hormone that is added to your IV drip to make the
contractions stronger and regular. This method is usually combined
with **ARM**. Although very safe, there are some risks and you will need
to be continually monitored after it has been administered. When
using syntocinon, contractions may be much more painful, stronger
and with shorter intervals between them as compared with those
started by natural labor.

LABOR

Bleeding during contractions

As labor progresses and the cervix opens, some women lose
small amounts of blood. This is generally nothing to worry about —
provided it is not associated with a low-lying placenta, abnormal
pain, or fetal distress. The amount of blood varies from woman to
woman. Some lose none at all, some lose a few streaks, and a few
lose enough to soak a pad. This blood loss is often a welcome sign
of progress. A skilled midwife is well able to assess the situation
and decide if the bleeding is normal or abnormal.

Epidurals

An epidural is a local anesthetic that is injected into the space
between your spinal column and spinal cord. This numbs the nerves
to the lower part of the body (stomach, back passage, vagina),
including the legs. As a result, you don't feel any pain in that part
of your body.

A mobile or low-dose epidural gives excellent pain relief but also
allows you to retain some sensation in your legs. However, you have
to remember that the primary aim of this kind of epidural is to relieve
pain; keeping you mobile is only a secondary concern, and some
women find that they're not really mobile at all. A mobile epidural
is set up in the same way as an ordinary epidural.

Epidurals can increase the length of labor, especially the pushing
stage. You might not be able to push completely because of lack of
sensation in that part of the body and a little assistance may be
required in delivering your baby.

It is worth pointing out that the success rate with epidurals is not
always 100% and midwives may prefer not to administer one if your
labor is progressing well, as there are risks (e.g., increasing length of
labor, lowering blood pressure).

Show

Either before labor starts, or early in labor, the plug of mucus
in the cervix, which has helped to seal the womb during pregnancy,
comes away and out of the vagina. This small amount of sticky pink
mucus is called a "show" – it's generally a mixture of blood and
mucus, typically with streaks or drops of bright red blood in a blob of
thick white or off-white mucus. This is perfectly normal and is usually
a welcome sign that labor may start in the next few hours or days
(although it may not start for a couple of weeks).

BIRTH

First stage of labor

This is the longest stage, usually lasting 6 to 10 hours. It can even last
up to 18 hours for a first baby. For second and subsequent babies it
usually lasts between 2 and 10 hours. During the first stage of labor,
your cervix will dilate and thin out to allow the baby to pass through
the birth canal. When you have reached ten centimeters dilation,
you know that your baby is ready to be born. This is the end of the
first stage.

Transitional stage

The transitional stage at the end of the first stage of labor can
be difficult, as you may be quite uncomfortable and yet not allowed
to push. You may shiver or tremble and some women experience
nausea or vomiting. Use the breathing techniques you have learned,
and try varying your position to make things a little easier.

Second stage

The second stage begins when your cervix is fully dilated. It generally lasts between 30 minutes and two hours for a first baby, and between ten minutes and one hour for a subsequent baby. During this stage, you actively push your baby through the birth canal.

Third stage

The third stage of labor begins after your baby is born and ends when the placenta, cord and membranes have been delivered. It usually takes less than half an hour. As your baby is being born, you might be given an injection of **oxytocin**. This hormone preparation helps the womb to contract and expel the placenta. **Syntocinon** or syntometrine are sometimes given to reduce the risk of excessive blood loss but this will depend on hospital policy and your choice.

Nausea/vomiting during labor
See **transitional stage**.

Second labors

It is thought that second labors are quicker because you know what to expect and are more relaxed and able to let your body get on with it. Also, your body has been physically "stretched" once before and so can do it more easily next time around.

Vacuum delivery

A ventouse delivery is an assisted delivery using a vacuum extractor. Your doctor or midwife may suggest a vacuum delivery during the second or pushing stage of labor for any of the following reasons.

* Your baby's head is not moving down through the pelvis (this is called "failure to progress").
* An epidural has relaxed your pelvic floor muscles too much, making it more difficult for your baby's head to make the right movements during the second stage.

* You are very tired.
* You need help to deliver a second twin.

Post-partum bleeding

After giving birth, whether by vaginal delivery or caesarean, you will experience moderate vaginal bleeding and discharge for the first two or three days. Initially, the blood will be red but this will subside to a brownish discharge called "lochia" and this may last up to six weeks. You should only use sanitary pads, never tampons (due to risk of infection).

Postpartum depression

At least half of all new mothers will experience what's known as the "baby blues." This is the most common form of depression and generally doesn't last long. After the initial high of giving birth, your milk comes in on or around the third day and this generally coincides with the onset of the blues: feeling tearful or irritable and quite low for reasons that you can't understand. There is no medical intervention as it's not a serious condition and will soon go away by itself! However, the ordinary stresses of motherhood, for some women, can turn into postpartum depression – it affects around 1 in 10 new mothers and usually does need to be treated. The BBC website (www.bbc.co.uk/health) suggests that the following may contribute to postpartum depression: insecurity and fear of abandonment, low self-esteem, feeling that the baby is more important than the mother, that a mother has become a slave to her baby, that freedom has been sacrificed and that the reality of being a mother comes as a bit of a shock. Men can also be affected by PND if they feel unable to cope or that they aren't giving the mother all the support she needs. It's important to try and recognize the symptoms as early as possible and go and see your doctor.

Pelvic floor exercises

The pelvic floor is made up of layers of muscle that support your uterus, bowel and bladder. Pregnancy and childbirth put pressure on these muscles, with the result that you might find yourself accidentally leaking pee when you sneeze, or cough. In order to stop this happening you can do exercises to tone up the pelvic floor muscles – they can be done at any time of the day, wherever you are, because all you have to do is simply pull in and tense your pelvic floor muscles as if you are stopping your flow of pee (although don't do this while you're actually in the bathroom having a pee!). Hold for a few seconds, then relax. If you aim to do small sets of repetitions throughout the day you should notice a difference, and no more leaks!

BREASTFEEDING

Breastfeeding helps the uterus return to its pre-pregnancy size after the birth. The release of oxytocin as the baby starts to feed encourages the uterus to contract.

Engorgement

During the first week after you give birth, you may find that your breasts feel very swollen, tender, throbbing, lumpy and uncomfortably full. Sometimes the swelling extends all the way to the armpit. You may have a temperature, too. Don't worry – as terrible as it sounds, this is truly a temporary, albeit painful, situation. It is caused by an abundance of breast milk becoming available to your baby. As that happens, more blood flows to your breasts, and some of the surrounding tissue swells. Try to remember that engorgement is a positive sign: you are producing milk to feed your baby, and soon, with the baby's help, you'll produce the right amount.

Foremilk and hindmilk

The foremilk is the breast milk the baby receives at the beginning of his or her feed. It comes primarily from a reservoir immediately behind the nipple so that there is a supply readily available for a hungry baby at the beginning of the feed. It is ample in quantity but less calorific than the hindmilk that follows.

In order for your baby to fully benefit from both these types of milk provided by your breasts, he or she needs to feed for a reasonable length of time. In the early days of breastfeeding, unrestricted feeding will ensure that your baby quickly regains his or her birth weight and sets up a good supply-and-demand system that will meet all his or her nutritional needs.

Let-down reflex

When you are breastfeeding your baby you will probably notice that, after he or she has been sucking for a few minutes, there is a strong tingling sensation in your breasts. This is the sensation of the let-down reflex which makes the milk ducts in the breast contract, squirting the milk out through the nipple.

It is your baby's sucking that stimulates the secretion of the hormone oxytocin, responsible also for the contractions of your womb during labor. While there is enough milk in the reservoir directly behind the nipple to meet your baby's immediate needs (the **foremilk**), the let-down reflex is essential to release the milk further back in the breast tissue (the **hindmilk**).

You may find that you notice this tingling sensation on other occasions, perhaps if you hear your baby cry, or as his or her normal feeding time approaches. You may also find that this is accompanied by some degree of leakage from the breasts. This may happen quite dramatically on one side when you are feeding your baby from the other, especially at first, but it should soon settle down as your milk production and feeding patterns become more closely synchronized.

Mastitis

Mastitis means, literally, inflammation of the breast. When mastitis occurs during breastfeeding, it is probably caused by a poor feeding technique or an ill-fitting bra. It is usually characterized by a wedge-shaped area of inflammation which feels tender and warm and looks red. Continuing to feed – having removed the bra and checked the position of the baby on the breast – will help the problem resolve itself quite quickly. If you become **engorged**, take steps to deal with it so that it doesn't give rise to mastitis.

If you don't continue to breastfeed with mastitis, the blockage that gave rise to the inflammation in the first place provides an ideal breeding ground for infection – and that could, in the worst case, give rise to a breast abscess. Infection can sometimes arise because the nipple has become sore and allowed access to infection. Sore nipples will usually only happen if your baby isn't latched on properly, or is positioned badly. Ask your midwife for advice, or contact your local breastfeeding counselor either from the La Leche League or hospital.

Diet during breastfeeding

During the whole time I was breastfeeding, Jamie was concerned that I was eating the wrong things and that it would affect both the baby and me. But the thing is, I didn't feel like eating. For him it was a practical issue that I should eat well and so he would get annoyed if I didn't. He was keen that I eat more healthily, and he would make lots of fish dishes for me (which I did actually love) to enrich my milk supply. I was concerned that I wasn't drinking enough water though. When Poppy was two weeks old I didn't seem to have enough milk in my breasts. The midwife said that the three things I should do were to get enough rest, eat well and drink lots of fluids. So I tried to drink about two quarts a day – it seemed to help as my milk supply increased and I also felt less tired.

WEANING

Many experts now recommend exclusive breastfeeding for the first six months but if you feel your baby needs to start solids before this then you should talk to your pediatrician. When it comes to moving on to cow's milk the recommended age is when your child is one.

SIDS

A few babies die every year unexpectedly and suddenly in their cribs. This is known as crib death or Sudden Infant Death syndrome. Although there is no clear explanation, a few precautions are known to reduce the risk of crib deaths:

* Always put babies to sleep on their backs as this is regarded as the safest position by doctors.
* Place your baby in the "feet-to-foot" position in the crib; your baby's feet should touch the end of the crib. Tuck covers in tight at the end of the crib and pull them up no higher than your baby's chest.
* Don't let your baby get too hot or too cold.
* Don't allow anyone to smoke around your baby or near the baby's room.
* Don't use a pillow for under twos as this could smother them.
* Remove all packaging from the mattress.

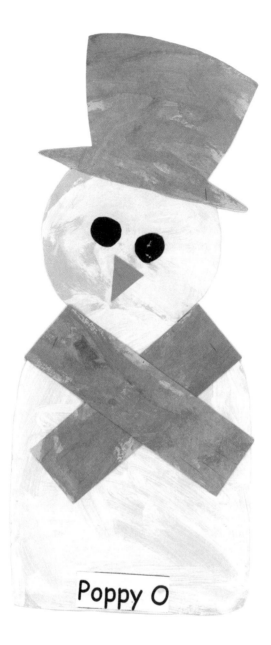

Poppy O

For more information on any of these topics,
check out the following websites:

www.b4baby.com

www.babycentre.co.uk

www.babydirectory.com

www.babyworld.co.uk

www.bbc.co.uk/health

www.boots.com

www.bounty.com

www.familiesonline.co.uk

www.huggies.com

www.mothercare.co.uk

www.mothersbliss.co.uk

www.netdoctor.co.uk

www.nhsdirect.nhs.uk

www.pampers.co.uk

http://parenting.ivillage.com

www.pregnancy.org

www.sofeminine.co.uk

www.storknet.com

www.ukparents.co.uk

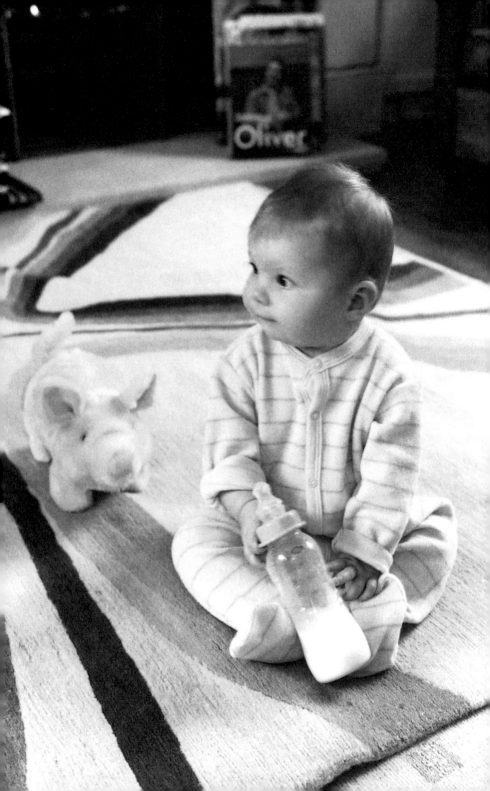

Things You Will Need

I thought this section might come in handy if you are preparing
for your first baby. Magazines and advertising for all kinds of different
things will hit you head-on and you'll be made to think that you are
going to have to buy every single bit of equipment there is . . . the
good news is that you don't have to. Here is a list of the things that
you probably will need, with notes on how I got along with them all.
I hope it helps.

BEDS AND BEDDING

Moses basket or bassinette
You may decide to put your newborn straight into a crib but I had
both my girls by the side of our bed in a basket for the first few weeks.
This meant that I could get to them right away when they woke for
feeding, although newborns are fairly loud in their sleep so if you
don't want to be disturbed by snuffles this may not work for you.

Cribs
I didn't know much about cribs – all I knew was that I wanted a
white one, so that helped to narrow down my search a bit. One of
the first things you will have to decide is whether or not you want
a crib or a crib bed. Crib or toddler beds are slightly bigger and will
see your baby through to about 5 years old, so they are economical as
you won't have to spend out for a separate bed when they outgrow
the crib. Of course, by this time you may have another baby so you
will have to buy a bed for your eldest and let the baby have the crib.

Bedding and Grobags (winter and summer)

I made a typical new mum mistake here and bought far too much bedding which I just didn't end up using. All you will probably need is a few sheets to go over the mattress and then sheets and blankets (for the first few months) followed by a Grobag. These are brilliant things which I used for both Poppy and Daisy. They are like miniature sleeping bags with arm holes and they do up with snaps (or zips for older children). This means that they can never wriggle out of them or end up with their head under the covers.

TRAVEL

Strollers

Before I had Poppy I had no idea that there were so many different types of carriages and strollers on the market. There are just so many options thrown at you and it can all become quite confusing. You need to know the sort of thing that you're going to want to use the stroller for most – if you go walking a lot in the countryside your best bet is an all-terrain one with big wheels, or you might want one that has a car seat which clicks on to it if you use your car a lot. I decided to buy a big traditional stroller with "venture" wheels as I thought this would be good for going out walking. I soon found out this was a Big Mistake though, as it was so heavy to push. So I then tried out a "3-in-1 travel system" with a car seat, which clicks on to the stroller for ease of getting baby in and out of the car without waking him or her up!

A lightweight stroller is ideal for when baby is a little bit older. These are great and you can pick up fairly cheap ones which will have everything you need in terms of a reclining back, swivel wheels or a net basket underneath for all your shopping! These are much lighter and easier to transport so it may even be good to have this kind of stroller as your main one and then buy a separate car seat which can be used from birth and then turned around when your baby is older.

Car seat

We bought a car seat that clicked onto a base unit in the car as well as clicking onto the stroller. This worked well, but next time around I might think about buying a separate car seat, which can be used from birth until age 3 or 4. These are usually backward-facing to start with, and then turned around when the baby weighs enough.

Travel bed

Obviously it depends on how much you're going to be away, but these are handy even at home as they can double up as a playpen.

Baby sling

These are fantastic for taking a younger baby out with you to the shops, or for a walk. We bought a brand called Baby Bjorn but there are lots of great ones on the market so have a look around. It's worth trying on different ones in the shop to see how easy they are to put on and also to see how they feel, as they all fit differently on your back and shoulders.

Diaper bag

An absolute must from Day One! You will probably find this will be one of the most-used of all your baby items. Don't go for a huge one in the first instance, even though it will seem like you need to take absolutely everything out with you, even if you're going food shopping! Get one that is big enough to hold a few diapers, a change of clothes, maybe a book or two, some burp cloths, wipes, and a changing mat. Separate pockets for bottles are worth looking out for, as are separate compartments for holding essentials like bottles of medicine, or travel-size tubes or jars of diaper cream.

CLOTHING

Undershirts and sleepers
I found that six short-sleeved undershirts and six onesies were enough to be going on with. I must admit that my two wore the onesies out and about until they were about six months old! Don't concern yourself with buying too many flashy baby clothes – you'll probably be given quite a few outfits and, also, you'll probably find it's so much easier to keep them in onesies! I can't deny they look cute in outfits though!

BATHING, FEEDING AND CHANGING

Bathing and cleaning essentials
For newborns all you will need are some cotton balls and maybe a little baby bath or a little container for water. You won't need any products for the first few months as their skin is so delicate; just use warm water and cotton or a soft washcloth.

Baby bath – I used one until the girls were five or six months old. To save your back, it might be worth getting one that has side grooves which fit over the edges of the bathtub so you don't have to bend right over. Anything to make life a little easier!

Plastic changing mat – any type of mat will do but padded ones are good. It is also worth putting a towel over it so your baby doesn't have to lie on the cold plastic.

Changing tables – I always found it easiest to change the girls on the floor but changing tables are good, especially for tiny babies who can't roll off.

Big bottle of baby lotion – always worth having as babies can get very dry skin.

Big tube of diaper cream – again, an essential which I'm sure most mothers of small children have in the house! Great for soothing diaper rash and other skin irritations. Have a big tube in the house and a smaller one for your out and about bag.

Diaper disposal bags – now, you may prefer to get one of those diaper bins with the scented liner inside but I preferred to always put dirty diapers in their own separate scented bags and then add them to the daily trash so they weren't hanging around. Either way, it's always worth having a supply of diaper disposal bags on hand.

Wipes – a total necessity, especially when your baby gets a little older and you can start to use cleansing things other than water on his or her skin. We can never have enough of these in the house, car, or diaper bag!

Other bits and bobs worth having are nail clippers, a forehead thermometer, infant Tylenol (acetaminophen) and Mylicon (for colic).

Diapers
The answer I found is to stock up with lots! I chose to go with disposable ones, although there are some great washable ones around these days (especially the organic brands like Kushies). Not knowing whether one brand was better than another, I tried Pampers Newborns first off but then found that Huggies Supreme were brilliant for keeping poos in place as they're elasticated well!

Burp cloths
I cannot stress how handy these squares of material are! I can't imagine motherhood without them! When the girls were tiny I used them during breastfeeding to catch any excess milk, or over my shoulder when burping after feeding. Babies will "posset" and bring up milky vomit after a feed and these cloths are perfect for wiping up any mess. They soon became used as comforters by Poppy and Daisy and they will nearly always have one near to hand.

Bibs

Not much to say about bibs really, other than you will need to get a stash of them. Like burp cloths, they are handy for newborns, especially after nursing.

Baby monitor

Good if you're not in earshot of the baby's room, if you're going to stay at a friend's house or if you're having an evening barbecue, etc. We also treated ourselves to a video baby monitor – brilliant for toddlers because you get to see what they're saying and doing when they're on their own in their bedrooms. Very funny!

RELAXATION

Baby bouncer

A great piece of equipment for babies before they can sit up on their own. I would put Poppy and Daisy into a bouncer chair and they would often fall asleep in it when they were tiny. This means that you can keep them in the same room as you to keep an eye on them during their nap, or you can transfer them easily to their crib. If I had to nip into the other room for something I knew that they would be safe in their bouncer chair. I also think they found it quite soothing to be gently rocked. You can actually buy these chairs with a built-in rocking facility but some babies don't like the vibrating sensation as much as being gently rocked. Easy to do with your foot while watching television!

FOR MUM

Breast pump
Essential if you decide to breastfeed. I bought a hand-held one,
but found it tiring and ineffective. However, the automatic one was
brilliant, and came in very useful, especially if you want your partner
to be involved in feeding the baby as it means that they can give the
baby a bottle. Some women prefer to express their milk by hand,
without using a pump at all, but this can be time-consuming and
a little tricky.

Tens machine
If you've never heard of one of these, they are basically hand-held
control packs with four pads attached. The pads can be stuck on
to your lower back and then you can control a small electric current
to pass through them into your back – it's a great distraction for
smaller contractions. It's not completely necessary to buy one of
these (as you can rent them as well) but I found it a great help in
the early stages of labor. I would say it's worth getting hold of one and
putting it in your labor bag, if only to pass the time away during those
arduous first hours of labor.

Gel-filled pads
I really didn't think that these would be necessary but I was so
pleased I did buy them because I used them over and over again
with both children. They are pads which can be chilled or warmed
up and placed over your breasts (as I did when I had mastitis)
or for putting on your bits down below after giving birth, to help
relieve the swelling.

THINGS YOU THINK YOU WILL NEED ...
BUT YOU'LL PROBABLY ONLY USE THEM
ONCE OR NOT AT ALL!

Swinging cradle
I don't deny that these look beautiful, but they really won't last you all that long and then you're stuck with a piece of furniture that you probably paid a lot of money for. For newborns I would suggest it's much better (and cheaper) to go with a Moses basket on a stand and then transfer them straight into their crib.

Swinging chair
Don't get drawn in by these things! Yes, they will probably get your baby off to sleep but you then run the risk of them only wanting to go to sleep in the chair, so I wouldn't waste any money on one. A bouncy chair is so much better I think.

Tons of bedding
As I said above, I only used fitted crib sheets to cover the mattress and then I used Grobags instead of sheets and blankets.

Big starter kit of toiletries
Don't get drawn in by the smell of these things!

Changing table
So much safer to change diapers on the floor, but if you would prefer to be upright then try a changing table with sides. Cheaper as well.

Newborn "all you need" packs
Don't succumb to the packages of scratch mittens, booties, hats to match, sleepsuits, etc – you won't use them! I thought it was a great idea but I think my girls only wore their scratch mittens a couple of times. And the hats never . . .

Diaper bin
Some mums love to use these but I never took mine out of the box it came in! Depends on how often you change your trash cans. If it's once a day then it might be best, as I did, to put each dirty diaper in a scented diaper disposal bag.

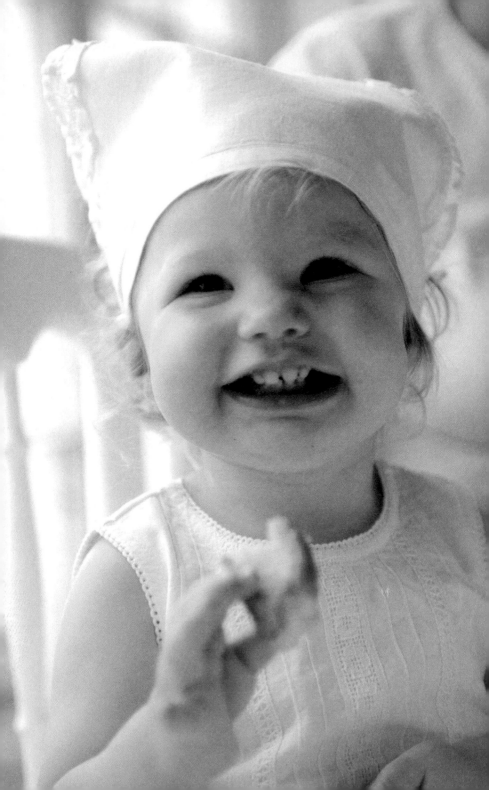

Where I Buy Baby Clothes

It's always fun to daydream about dressing your new baby up in the cutest clothes. I'm already looking forward to taking my two girls out on fun shopping trips when they're older!

I had been given quite a few baby clothes before Poppy was born and I had stored quite a lot away in case it was bad luck to have more of one sex's clothing! But nearer my due date I allowed myself to buy all the essential little white onesies, booties and hats to put in the nursery. Ever since I was a little girl I have had a definite idea as to how I wanted to dress my children. With both my girls I dressed them in snow white cotton onesies until they were at least six months old. All my NCT girlfriends were horrified that I had not yet introduced Poppy to a three-piece outfit, and to think that I had a girl – they saw it as almost a crime that she was not sitting pretty in a little floral number with ribboned booties! But I just felt that little babies should stay little babies for as long as they can, as all too soon they grow up.

My mum had promised that I could inherit all the baby clothes that my sisters and I wore if I had girls, as my older sister has had all boys . . . so far, I have inherited everything and I love all of it – it's what is called vintage now! I really like the idea of dressing the girls in quite old-fashioned floral dresses, angel tops, frilly underpants and dungarees. So I was pretty much set for clothes for the first year. But that didn't stop me buying some more modern outfits! Poppy would sleep contentedly in the baby carrier whilst I wandered around Baby Gap hanging various garments off the Baby Bjorn to see if they might fit her/suit her! I was very pleased to see that she was enjoying these little shopping trips, but then again she was only five weeks old and fast asleep most of the day anyway! It wasn't until she reached about 18 months that her shopping phobia began . . . I would either grin and bear the embarrassment of her tantrums or pass right by without stopping – it all depends on how I'm feeling and, these days, whether Daisy decides to have a tantrum at the same time.

Now, I know that not all of these places have set up shop outside Britain, but I wanted to share some of my favorites anyway. My favorite shops to buy Poppy and Daisy's clothes from are:

Baby Gap
The obvious; because it's just around the corner from where we live and it does have clothes for girls. If you search carefully you can get things which you may not always see on other children and you can mix them with other pieces from other shops for added quirkiness. Their sale rack usually has some fab stuff on it as well. For Poppy's second birthday I bought her the sweetest white broderie anglaise dress there and customized it with a thick cream ribbon sash from John Lewis. Set off with tights, little white Mary Jane shoes and a striped blazer she looked like she'd just stepped off the set of *Mary Poppins* – fantastic!

Mini Boden and other catalogues
For really special occasions, I love searching through catalogues for their clothes as you can usually find something different. My favorite one is Mini Boden – they also do lovely boys' clothes, according to my sister. Little Gems is a really sweet catalogue, although mainly for very young babies. They sell old-fashioned, fresh, white cotton appliqué dresses which are very cute.

H&M
These two shops are brilliant as they are both really reasonably priced. The clothes are traditional but they also offer more funky pieces.

Boutiques

Without wanting to sound like I have just stepped out of the London School of Fashion, if I really want to treat the girls (which actually means treating me as Daisy certainly wouldn't mind if she had to wear a boiler suit every day; as long as she can roll around in the mud she is happy!) I love the more independent boutiques such as Their Nibs in Notting Hill, or notsobig in Highgate. Both of these shops have real one-of-a-kind pieces and lovely traditional shoes and accessories.

Other than that, it's back to the hand-me-downs from my mum! These are actually the outfits that are always commented on by my friends. The old ones are always the best. I'm definitely not into designer labels for children. For starters, I find the prices absolutely ridiculous and don't see the point in spending that much for something that the girls will grow out of in just three months. I also think it's awful to see children dressed in clothing with the designer's name emblazoned across it – that's all just too much too young and, frankly, most of the designer styles are far too grown up for the girls. High-heeled boots at the age of two . . . NO THANK YOU!

Having said that, just the other day, when the girls were playing in my bedroom, I suddenly realized that it had gone very quiet. I peeped around the door and saw that they had emptied out my entire shoe cupboard. Poppy was wandering round the room in my pink silk round-toed high heels (my favorites), holding a little silver clutch bag. Daisy, typically, had chosen to put on my battered cowboy boots (which reached up to her hips) and she was chanting "Woody, Woody, Buzz!" GIRLS!! Thank goodness I have control over what they wear now as I can already hear myself saying, "You are not going out like that!"

Here is a run down of places that I shop at for the girls:

Top five Main Street shops – Baby Gap, H&M, Petit Bateau, Monsoon

Top five catalogues – Mini Boden, Little Gems, Mitty James, Blooming Marvellous, Urchin (great for outer wear – raincoats, wellies, etc)

Top five boutiques – Rachel Riley in Marylebone High Street (really traditional outfits like smock tops), Their Nibs in Notting Hill (vintage clothing and their own label), Look Who's Walking in Heath Street, Hampstead (the clothes are designer, but the shoes are lovely and traditional); notsobig in Highgate; Cheeky Monkeys in Notting Hill (nice pajamas!)

Top five places for gifts – Urchin (brilliant for presents and also for things like flags or party bags), The Great Little Trading Company, Letterbox (good for traditional wooden toys and personalized gifts), Bohemia in Regents Park Road, Humla in Flask Walk, Hampstead (really interesting gifts and lovely staff)

Department stores are always great because you get everything under one roof so you can have a really good browse. I tend to go to John Lewis if there's one nearby. For buying basics like undershirts, onesies and T-shirts, I go to shops like Woolworths or Primark. Good supermarkets now have baby sections that are great value for money.

And here are some websites which are worth taking a look at:

www.babygap.com

www.bloomingmarvellous.co.uk

www.cathkidston.co.uk

www.gltc.co.uk

www.jigsaw-online.com

www.letterbox.co.uk

www.petitbateau.co.uk

www.theirnibs.com

www.urchin.co.uk

www.wingreen.co.uk

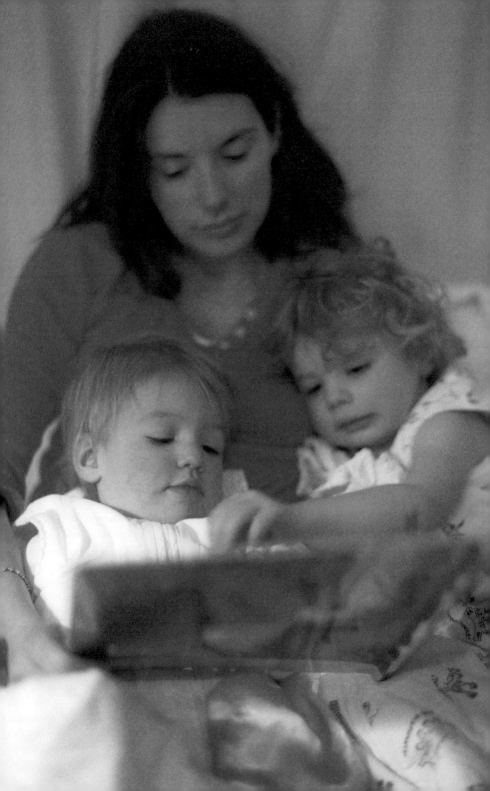

Books That I found Useful

Annabel Karmel food books
I like all Annabel's books – I find that I dip into them for recipes. She
was the first author I read about weaning as she gives great advice.

Pregnancy the Natural Way by Zita West
(Dorling Kindersley, 0 751 327573, 2001)
I found this very useful – it gives lots of practical information
about complementary therapies for pregnancy, to natural pain
relief in labor.

Secrets of the Baby Whisperer by Tracy Hogg with Melinda Blau
(Vermilion, 0 091 857023, 2001)
This is a fantastic book if you fancy introducing some sort of routine
into your baby's life, but you don't want to be too regimented or
strict. It's like the softer version of Gina Ford and I really liked it.

The Complete Book of Baby Names (Traditional and Modern)
by Hilary Spence
(Foulsham Publishing House, 0 572 026676, 2001)
This is a pretty good reference book for names. I definitely found
some possibles for our two children had they been boys,
so I will save these ideas for the future!

The Girlfriends' Guide to Surviving the First Year of Motherhood
by Vicki Iovine
(Penguin Group (USA), 0 747 533253, 1997)
This is a fab book and completely different to what I had been
reading. It's very funny and I found myself racing downstairs to

read sections out to Jamie, knowing that he would understand and empathize along with me. Hilarious in parts!

The Miraculous World of Your Unborn Baby by Nikki Bradford
(Salamander Books Ltd., 1 840 652527, 2001)
Jamie bought this book for me as he knew how absolutely fascinated I was (and still am) with the miracle of birth. It is fantastic to see just how amazing the birth process is. Brilliant.

Complete Baby and Childcare by Dr. Miriam Stoppard
(Dorling Kindersley, 0 751 312339, 2001)
The classic – everyone should have a copy! A huge book, filled to the brim with everything you could ever want to know!

Johnson's Child Development: Your Baby from Birth to Six Months
(Dorling Kindersley, 0 751 33717X, 2002)

Johnson's Child Development: Your Baby from Six to Twelve Months
(Dorling Kindersley, 0 751 337188, 2002)
I just stumbled across these books when I was bored one afternoon. I took Poppy out in her baby sling and went to sit in Waterstones – this was about as far as my entertainment went at that point! The books are fab as they explain the development process simply and it's great to see if your baby is "on track." They are very easy to read – just what you need after a hard day's mummying!

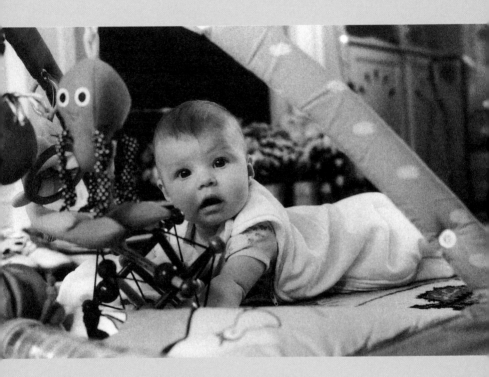

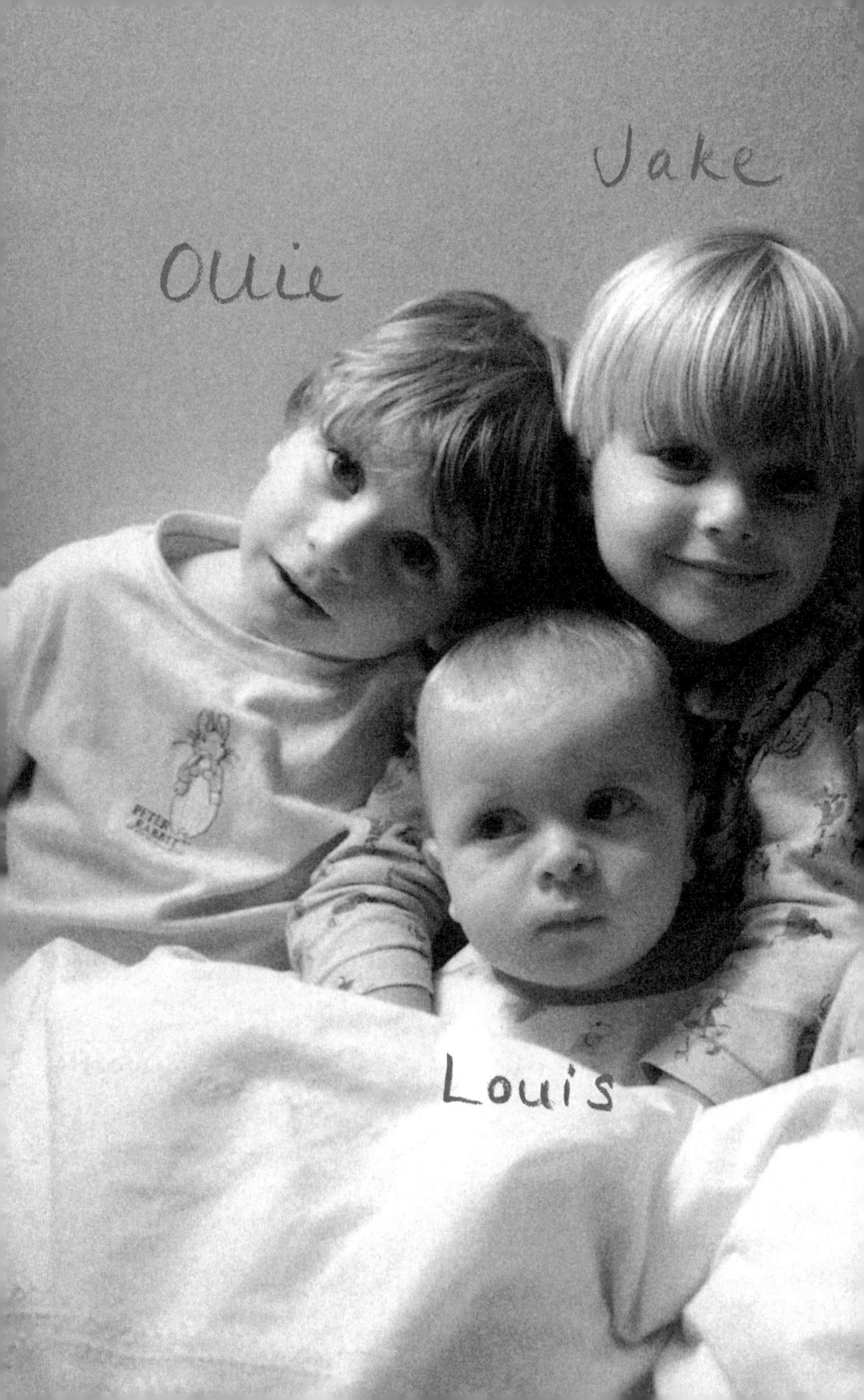
Jake
Ollie
Louis

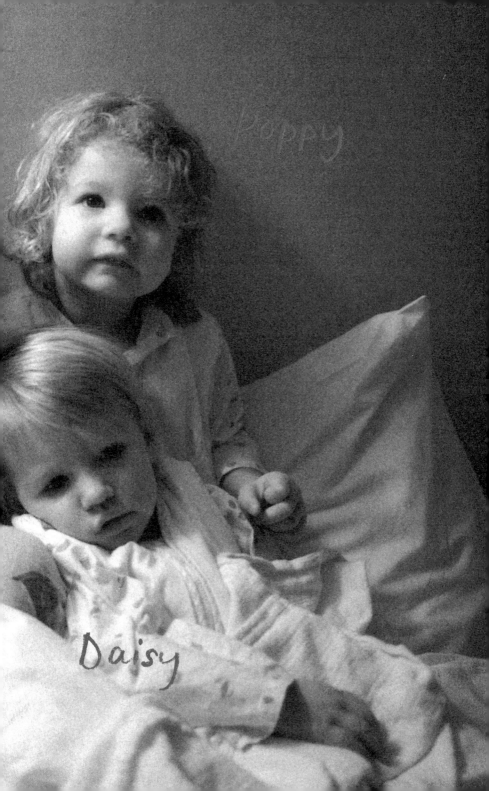

Poppy

Daisy

THANKS

So many thank yous and big appreciations go to:

My hero, Mr. Geoffrey Trew – my gynecologist from Queen
Charlotte's and Chelsea Hospital. Without his expertise, knowledge
and gentle kindness I am not sure we would have our precious girls
now. Also a big thank you for assisting me with all the medical bits
in the book.

Dr. Andrew McCarthy, my obstetrician and the man who delivered
both my babies. Thank you for your calmness, patience and general
brilliance at your job – roll on baby number three!

All the midwives and staff at Queen Charlotte's. Thank you
especially for taking my incessant calls during my pregnancy and
answering my many questions with tolerance and understanding.

My wonderful husband, Jamie – I love you so much. Thank you
for being the best daddy in the world and for feeding me delicious
food and massaging my feet while I tapped away on my computer.
And all the photos you took which have been used throughout the
book are fab – thanks! You are the BEST!

Our two beautiful daughters, Poppy and Daisy – you make us
laugh, you make us cry but most of all you complete our family
and make your Mummy and Daddy so very proud. We adore you.

To my amazing mum – thank you for ALWAYS, ALWAYS being
there for me. You are a constant support, a fantastic Granny and
someone I can really laugh with. My Saturday mornings wouldn't
be the same without our usual shopping trip to Cambridge followed
by a cappuccino in the car. I LOVE YOU.

To my sisters, Nathalie and Lisa, for being my best friends.
Thanks for your wonderful support. To my brother-in-law, Lionel,
and Lisa's boyfriend, Sal.

To the rest of my family – Trevor and Sally, my mum and dad-in-
law, for being fantastic grandparents; and to Anna-Marie and Paul
for being a lovely aunty and uncle. Thanks for all your brilliant

medical advice when it comes to my little girls, Anna. To all my
gorgeous little nephews – I love you all very much.

My best friend, Nix, just for being you. Love you lots.

A huge thanks to Lindsey Evans – my editor and God-mummy
to Pops – for spending countless hours making sense of my endless
paragraphs and checking through all my spelling mistakes! But
most of all for being a wonderful listener and a great friend to discuss
pointless magazine gossip with over tea and cake!

Louise Moore at Penguin – thanks for believing in me enough to
take this book on knowing that it was probably a complete gamble . . .
I hope that I can make you proud. Fancy a sequel?

Finally, a huge thank you to everyone who has been involved
in the process of publishing this book, especially all the guys at
Smith & Gilmour and the lovely John Hamilton for designing the
cover and all the cool bits inside.

Big thanks to all at Penguin who have helped to make this book
reach the shelves, especially Claire Bord, Jane Opoku, Sophie Brewer,
Naomi Fidler, Helen Reeve, Keith Taylor and Fiona Brown.

The very cool and trendy Chris Terry – thank you so much for
making our photo days such fun and for producing really fab
pictures. My girls love you.

For contributing to the photography – the lovely David Loftus,
Harry Borden and John Carey.

Thanks so much to Cath Kidston for the use of the rose on the
jacket and throughout the book.

All the guys at Jamie's office – especially Danny McCubbin for
being a great listener and a wonderful friend; Louise Holland, for
always being on the other end of the phone for me; and my lovely
friend Ginny Rolfe, for all her advice and support.

James and Nicky, for being wonderful friends and brilliant with
my girls.

And thanks to Ginny Brunton and Edward Sylvester for advice
on the medical bits and pieces – I appreciate it!

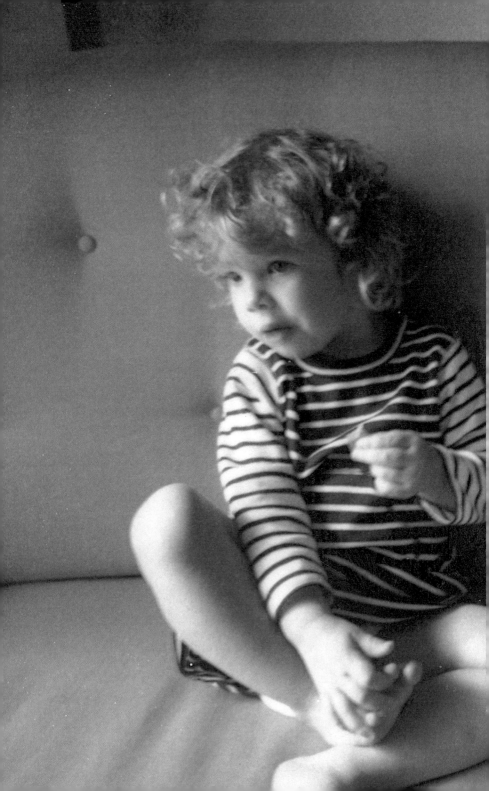

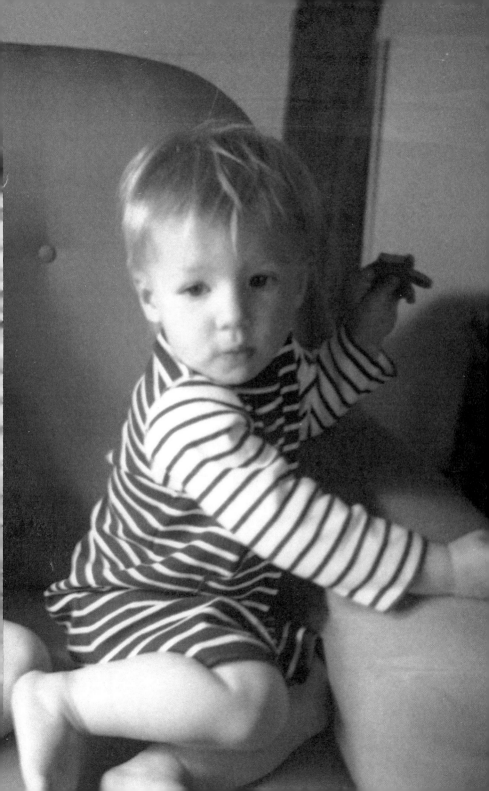

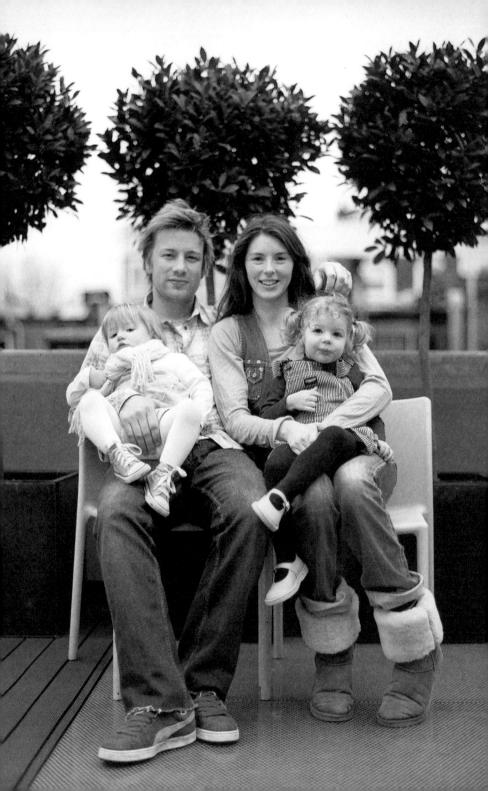

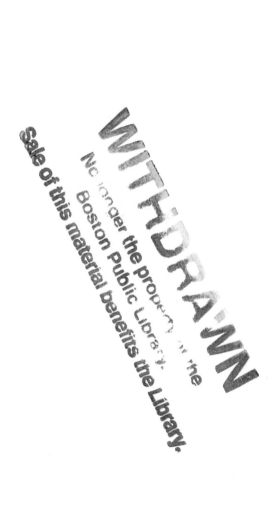

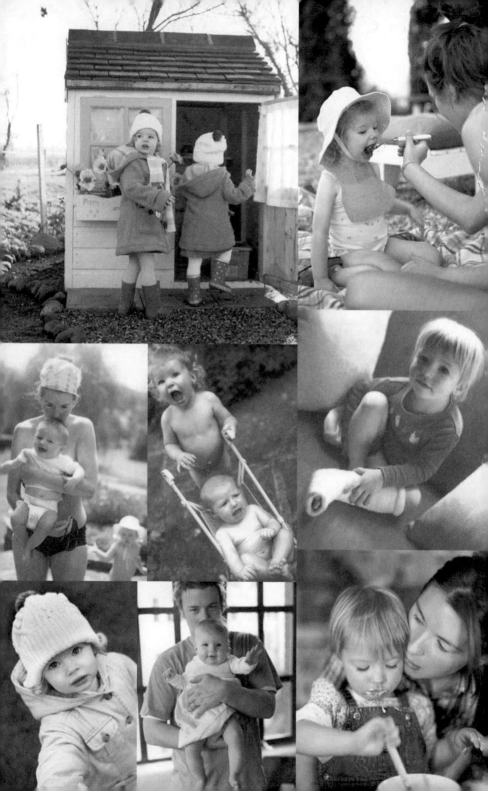